JOURNEY INTO NEI GONG, SHEN GONG AND NEI DAN

A COURSE IN INNER ALCHEMY

RICHARD CAASI

Copyright © 2025

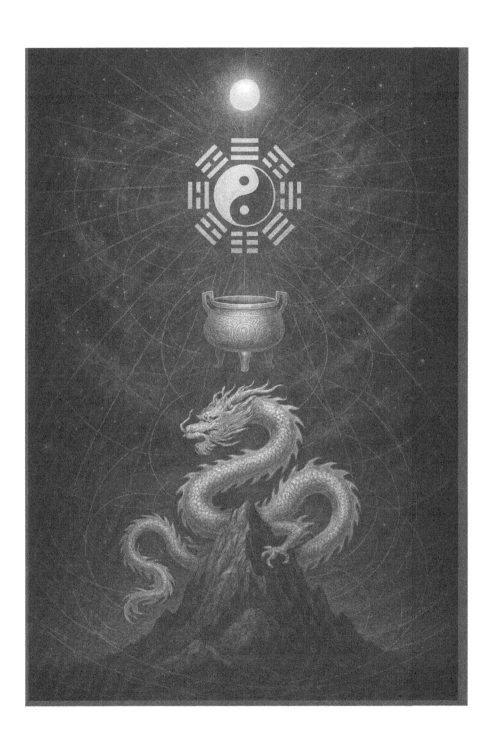

Table of Contents

Dedication

To all seekers walking the winding path of inner alchemy—
May your journey through dreams, breath, and stillness lead you ever inward,
To the golden light within,
Where the boundaries dissolve, the self transforms,
And the eternal reveals itself in silence.

This book is for you—
The quiet alchemists of the soul.

Disclaimer

The practices, techniques, and information presented in *A Journey Through Nei Gong, Shen Gong, and Taoist Internal Alchemy* are intended for educational and personal development purposes only. They are not intended to diagnose, treat, cure, or prevent any medical, psychological, or psychiatric condition.

Always consult with your physician, therapist, or other qualified healthcare provider before beginning any new exercise, breathwork, meditation, or energy practice—especially if you are pregnant, have a chronic health condition, or are under medical supervision.

While the author and contributors have made every effort to ensure the accuracy and safety of the practices shared in this book, they accept no responsibility for any outcome or injury resulting from the application of these teachings. Your health and well-being are your personal responsibility.

The internal cultivation methods described herein, including Nei Gong, Shen Gong, and Taoist Internal Alchemy, can involve intense personal transformation, energetic shifts, and emotional release. Proceed with awareness, discernment, and at your own pace. If you experience strong physical, emotional, or mental reactions, pause your practice and seek guidance from a qualified professional or teacher.

This work includes spiritual concepts and metaphysical interpretations that may not align with all belief systems. Readers are encouraged to take what resonates, leave what doesn't, and always follow their own inner guidance.

By engaging with the material in this book, you agree to hold the author, publisher, and any affiliated parties harmless from any and all liability related to your personal experience and practice.

Part 0 Preliminaries

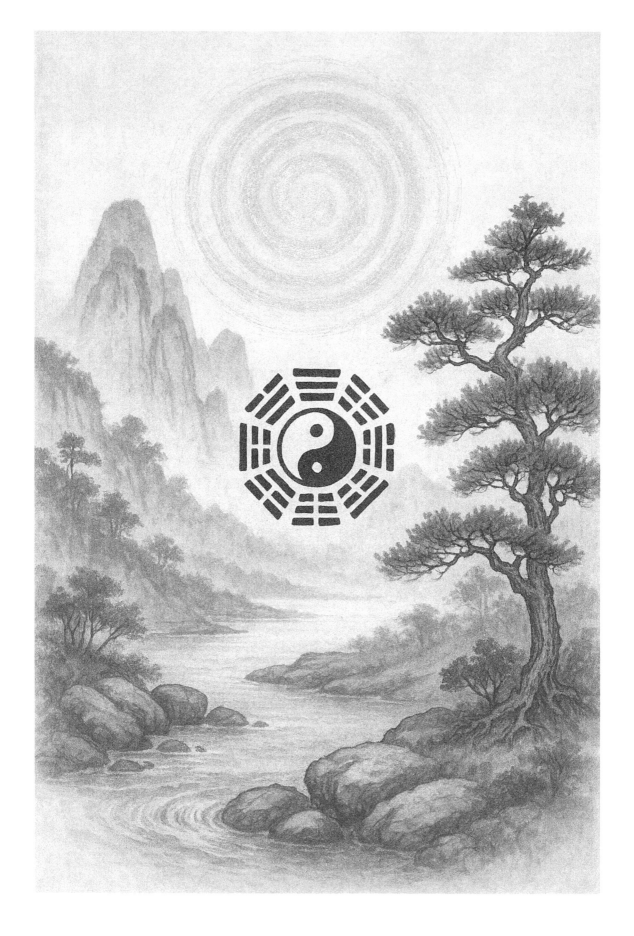

Welcome to a comprehensive journey through the ancient yet powerfully relevant arts of **Nei Gong**, **Shen Gong**, and **Taoist Internal Alchemy (Nei Dan)**. This book and course are designed to help you unlock your full inner potential—physically, energetically, mentally, and spiritually—through a step-by-step progression rooted in Taoist tradition and adapted for modern practitioners.

Whether you are a seasoned **Qigong practitioner**, a dedicated **energy healer**, a **biohacker**, an **athlete**, a **yoga teacher**, or someone newly curious about meditation and inner transformation, this program meets you exactly where you are—and gently guides you forward.

The Flow of the Journey

Taoist inner cultivation is not a random collection of techniques. It is a **natural progression**, a spiral path of returning to your original nature. This course flows through four progressive stages:

1. **Nei Gong** – Cultivating the body and energy
2. **Shen Gong** – Cultivating consciousness and spirit
3. **Internal Alchemy (Nei Dan)** – Refining the Three Treasures (Jing, Qi, Shen)
4. **Emptiness (Xu / Wuji)** – Returning to the Tao, beyond form

This structure follows the alchemical formula:

Jing → Qi → Shen → Xu → Tao

Each stage builds on the last—transforming dense essence into subtle awareness, then dissolving that awareness into emptiness. It's a process of refining, elevating, and ultimately transcending.

What You'll Learn

- **Foundational energy practices** to ground, balance, and circulate Qi
- **Breathwork and meditation** to activate Dantian centers
- **Alchemical visualizations and inner breath** to transmute energy
- **Awareness and witness cultivation** to awaken Shen
- **Techniques to experience Emptiness** and merge with the Tao

Each chapter includes:

- Clear, structured **explanations of theory**
- Simple yet powerful **daily practices**
- A **workbook** to track progress and reflect
- Practical integration into daily life

COURSE CURRICULUM: *A 12-Week Inner Alchemy Journey*

Week	Theme	Practices	Milestone
1	Setting Intentions + Energy Basics	Breath, posture, grounding	Awareness of body tension & energy flow
2	Dantian Activation	Belly breathing, energy ball	Feeling warmth or tingling in Dantian
3	Microcosmic Orbit	Orbit meditation, spinal awareness	Orbit flow sensation begins
4	Jing Cultivation & Vitality Boost	Jing hygiene, retention, herbs	Increased energy and clarity
5	Upper Dantian Activation	Shen breathing, inner light	Third eye pulsing or light vision
6	Observer Awareness	Noting practice, inner silence	Observing thoughts without identification
7	Heart-Mind Harmony	Heart meditation, Xin softening	Emotional resilience and coherence
8	Dreamwork + Spirit Contact	Dream recall, spirit visualization	Lucid dream or spiritual impression
9	Fusion Practices (Qi to Shen)	Five element fusion, Shen consolidation	Stable awareness beyond body-mind
10	Emptiness Practice (Wuji)	Formless meditation, inner stillness	Glimpses of formless presence
11	Tao in Life	Everyday mindfulness, inner listening	Flowing decisions and effortless action

Week	Theme	Practices	Milestone
12	Completion + Integration	Self-review, offering gratitude	Inner stability, unity, renewed direction

Who Is This For?

This program is designed to serve **diverse paths of mastery and healing**:

Qigong & Martial Arts Practitioners

- Deepen your understanding of Qi
- Amplify internal power and sensitivity
- Balance form with formless flow

Energy Healers (Reiki, Quantum Touch, etc.)

- Strengthen your energy body
- Improve discernment and energetic boundaries
- Clear channels for intuitive information

Meditation Practitioners & Yogis

- Move from passive meditation to energy refinement
- Explore subtle layers of awareness (Shen)
- Access states of stillness beyond thought

Biohackers & Longevity Enthusiasts

- Cultivate vitality from within (Jing and Qi preservation)
- Activate regenerative energy states
- Harmonize body, brain, and nervous system naturally

Athletes & Performers

- Improve physical coordination and recovery
- Train breath, focus, and internal power
- Tap into flow states and body intelligence

Spiritual Seekers & Mystics

- Follow a complete map of inner evolution
- Balance awakening with embodiment
- Connect directly to the Tao—within and without

Prerequisites

No previous experience in Taoist practice is required. However, a basic level of the following will help:

- An open mind and willingness to feel
- A few minutes of daily discipline
- A quiet place to practice when possible

If you already practice Qigong, yoga, meditation, or healing work, you'll find this system synergizes beautifully with your existing path. It adds structure and depth to subtle energies, internal perception, and spiritual integration.

The Benefits You Can Expect

With consistent and sincere practice, the following benefits naturally arise:

- Increased **vitality**, **grounding**, and **mental clarity**
- Greater **emotional stability** and **heart-centered presence**
- Heightened **intuition**, **dream recall**, and **spiritual vision**
- Deep connection to **nature**, **emptiness**, and the **Tao**
- A calm, spacious **awareness** that remains unshaken in life's chaos

How to Proceed

You can use this book in three ways:

1. **As a self-study course** (12-week or open-ended)
2. **As a personal practice companion** (build your own rhythm)
3. **As a teaching tool** (for instructors and group facilitators)

Each chapter includes theory, daily exercises, reflection prompts, and integration tips. A **Workbook** at the end of each chapter lesson and a **Practice Tracker and Journal** is provided to help you stay aligned and attentive to your growth.

A Journey Inward, A Return to Wholeness

This is not a race. This is a remembrance.

You are already whole, already connected to the Tao. These practices don't give you anything new—they remove what blocks you from seeing what is already present. Stillness, clarity, power, compassion, emptiness… they are already yours.

All you must do is return to them.

Let's begin.

Inner Alchemy Practice Tracker & Journal

Use this tracker to follow your Nei Gong, Shen Gong, and Internal Alchemy practice over 12 weeks. Reflect on your experiences and insights in the journal section below each week.

Weekly Practice Tracker

Week	Focus / Theme	Practices	Time Practiced (min/day)	Notes
Week 1	Setting Intentions + Energy Basics			
Week 2	Dantian Activation			
Week 3	Microcosmic Orbit			
Week 4	Jing Cultivation & Vitality			
Week 5	Upper Dantian Activation			
Week 6	Observer Awareness			
Week 7	Heart-Mind Harmony			
Week 8	Dreamwork + Spirit Contact			
Week 9	Fusion Practices (Qi to Shen)			

Week 10	Emptiness Practice (Wuji)			
Week 11	Tao in Life			
Week 12	Completion + Integration			

Use this space to record insights, energetic shifts, dreams, or spiritual messages received during practice.

Week 1: Setting Intentions + Energy Basics

What did I feel during practice?

What changed in my energy, awareness, or emotions?

What insights or dreams came through?

Other reflections:

Week 2: Dantian Activation

What did I feel during practice?

What changed in my energy, awareness, or emotions?

What insights or dreams came through?

Other reflections:

Week 3: Microcosmic Orbit

What did I feel during practice?

What changed in my energy, awareness, or emotions?

What insights or dreams came through?

Other reflections:

Week 4: Jing Cultivation & Vitality

What did I feel during practice?

What changed in my energy, awareness, or emotions?

What insights or dreams came through?

Other reflections:

Week 5: Upper Dantian Activation

What did I feel during practice?

What changed in my energy, awareness, or emotions?

What insights or dreams came through?

Other reflections:

Week 6: Observer Awareness

What did I feel during practice?

What changed in my energy, awareness, or emotions?

What insights or dreams came through?

Other reflections:

Week 7: Heart-Mind Harmony

What did I feel during practice?

What changed in my energy, awareness, or emotions?

What insights or dreams came through?

Other reflections:

Week 8: Dreamwork + Spirit Contact

What did I feel during practice?

What changed in my energy, awareness, or emotions?

What insights or dreams came through?

Other reflections:

Week 9: Fusion Practices (Qi to Shen)

What did I feel during practice?

What changed in my energy, awareness, or emotions?

What insights or dreams came through?

Other reflections:

Week 10: Emptiness Practice (Wuji)

What did I feel during practice?

What changed in my energy, awareness, or emotions?

What insights or dreams came through?

Other reflections:

Week 11: Tao in Life

What did I feel during practice?

What changed in my energy, awareness, or emotions?

What insights or dreams came through?

Other reflections:

Week 12: Completion + Integration

What did I feel during practice?

What changed in my energy, awareness, or emotions?

What insights or dreams came through?

Other reflections:

PART I: Foundations – Preparing the Vessel

The Three Treasures and the Path to Emptiness

The Ancient Path: From Nei Gong to Emptiness

At its core, Chinese internal cultivation follows a natural progression that has been refined over thousands of years. This journey moves from the tangible to the increasingly subtle, from physical to metaphysical, ultimately leading to a state that transcends all dualistic concepts.

Nei Gong represents the foundation of internal cultivation. Translating roughly to "internal skill" or "internal work," it encompasses practices that develop and refine the body's internal energy systems. These methods include specialized breathing techniques, physical postures, mental concentration exercises, and subtle movements designed to open energy pathways and strengthen the practitioner's vital essence. The body becomes the laboratory, where through careful attention and dedicated practice, one begins to sense and direct the flow of life force.

As the practitioner advances, Shen Gong practices become accessible. While Nei Gong primarily focuses on the body and energy, Shen Gong directs attention to the cultivation of spirit or consciousness. Here, the emphasis shifts from energy manipulation to the refinement of awareness itself. Meditation deepens, the mind becomes increasingly stable, and the practitioner begins to experience states of consciousness beyond ordinary perception. The boundary between self and other starts to become more permeable.

The alchemical phase represents a profound transformation where the practitioner begins the process of spiritual transmutation. Drawing from Taoist alchemical traditions, this stage involves the symbolic "cooking" of the internal essences to produce the "elixir of immortality." In practical terms, this means the systematic refinement and integration of the body's vital substances and energies to support elevated states of consciousness. The practitioner works with increasingly subtle energetic phenomena, learning to direct attention with extraordinary precision and developing the capacity to enter profound meditative absorptions.

Finally, the path culminates in Emptiness (Wu or Xu in Chinese traditions). This is not nihilistic nothingness but rather a state beyond conceptualization—the absolute reality from which all phenomena arise and to which they return. In emptiness, the practitioner realizes the fundamental nature of mind and existence. All dualistic thinking falls away, and one experiences direct communion with the Tao itself. This state transcends all descriptions but is characterized by boundless awareness, profound peace, and the spontaneous manifestation of wisdom and compassion.

The Three Treasures: Jing, Qi, Shen

At the heart of Taoist internal cultivation lies the concept of the Three Treasures—Jing, Qi, and Shen. These represent the fundamental substances or energies that comprise human existence, and their cultivation, preservation, and refinement form the basis of spiritual practice.

Jing (Essence) is the most tangible of the three treasures. Often described as the body's foundational substance, it governs physical development, reproduction, and overall vitality. In its most concentrated form, Jing is associated with reproductive fluids, but it actually permeates all tissues and organs. We receive prenatal Jing from our parents at conception, while postnatal Jing is acquired through food, air, and sensory impressions. Practices to preserve and refine Jing include proper diet, adequate rest, moderation in sexual activity, and specific Qi Gong exercises that stimulate the kidneys and endocrine system. The preservation of Jing is essential for longevity and forms the material basis for spiritual development.

Qi (Vital Energy) represents the dynamic, animating force that flows through all living things. Neither purely physical nor completely non-material, Qi occupies the middle ground between matter and energy. It circulates through the body's meridian system, vitalizing organs and tissues while facilitating communication between different bodily systems. Qi cultivation involves practices like regulated breathing, mindful movement, and meditation. As Qi becomes abundant and refined, it can transform denser Jing into more subtle energies, and in turn, be transformed into Shen. When Qi flows smoothly and abundantly, health flourishes, emotional balance prevails, and the mind becomes clear and focused.

Shen (Spirit) is the most refined of the three treasures. It encompasses consciousness, mental activity, and spiritual awareness. In its ordinary aspect, Shen manifests as clear thinking, emotional intelligence, and moral discernment. In its transcendent aspect, it represents the divine spark within—our connection to the Tao itself. Shen cultivation involves practices that quiet the mind, expand awareness, and cultivate virtuous qualities like compassion, wisdom, and integrity.

As Shen develops, the practitioner experiences increasing clarity, intuition, and spiritual insight.

The relationship between the Three Treasures is often described through alchemical metaphors: Jing is the raw material, Qi is the transformative fire, and Shen is the refined gold that results from the process. The treasures exist in a dynamic balance, each supporting and transforming into the others through proper cultivation. In advanced practice, they ultimately unify into what is sometimes called the "Golden Flower" or "Immortal Embryo"—a symbol of spiritual realization where the three treasures return to their unified source.

Wu Wei and Returning to the Tao

The concept of Wu Wei—often translated as "non-action" or "effortless action"—represents one of the most profound and paradoxical teachings in Taoist philosophy. Far from encouraging passivity or indifference, Wu Wei describes action that arises spontaneously from alignment with the Tao rather than from the striving of the ego-self.

In practical terms, Wu Wei manifests as action that feels natural, timely, and appropriate to the circumstances. It emerges when we have cultivated sufficient wisdom to recognize the inherent patterns and tendencies in situations, allowing us to respond with minimal interference. Like water flowing around obstacles rather than struggling against them, Wu Wei represents the path of least resistance that nevertheless accomplishes what is needed.

Within internal cultivation practices, Wu Wei appears in seemingly contradictory instructions: "Practice diligently, yet without striving." "Maintain awareness, yet allow the mind to settle naturally." "Guide the Qi, yet do not force it." These paradoxes point to the middle way between excessive effort and negligence that characterizes authentic practice. The practitioner learns to create the appropriate conditions for transformation and then allows the process to unfold according to its natural rhythm.

As cultivation deepens, Wu Wei becomes increasingly central. The practitioner realizes that the very effort to attain spiritual realization can become an obstacle if it reinforces the sense of a separate self striving for achievement. True advancement occurs when this separation begins to dissolve, and practice becomes less a matter of "doing" and more a process of "allowing" or "unveiling" what has always been present.

This brings us to the ultimate aim of all Taoist cultivation: returning to the Tao. The Tao Te Ching opens with the recognition that "the Tao that can be spoken is not the eternal Tao," acknowledging that our final destination transcends conceptual understanding. Yet the text also provides guidance for the journey of return, emphasizing qualities like simplicity, humility, compassion, and contentment.

Returning to the Tao means recognizing and harmonizing with our original nature—the unconditioned awareness that precedes all mental formations. It involves shedding accumulated layers of conditioning, conceptual thinking, and habitual patterns that obscure our inherent clarity. Like polishing a mirror to reveal its reflective capacity, we remove obstructions to allow our natural luminosity to shine forth.

This return is not a linear journey to an external destination but rather a spiraling process of awakening to what has always been present. As the Taoist sage Chuang Tzu noted, "The perfect man employs his mind as a mirror. It grasps nothing; it refuses nothing. It receives, but does not keep." In this mirror-like awareness, free from grasping and aversion, we discover that we have never truly been separate from the Tao.

The cultivation of the Three Treasures, the practice of Wu Wei, and the ultimate return to the Tao thus form a coherent and comprehensive path. Beginning with the tangible refinement of body and energy, proceeding through increasingly subtle states of consciousness, and culminating in the recognition of our fundamental nature, this journey leads from multiplicity back to unity, from complexity to sublime simplicity.

The Energetic Anatomy - Dantians, Meridians, and the Body-Mind-Spirit Integration

The human body is far more than mere flesh and bone. For millennia, Eastern healing traditions have recognized that we are animated and sustained by subtle energies that flow through specific pathways and collect in powerful centers throughout the body. This understanding forms the foundation of practices such as qigong, tai chi, acupuncture, and various meditation techniques that have endured through the ages. In this chapter, we will explore the three Dantians, the meridian system, and how these energetic structures create the bridge between body, mind, and spirit.

Unlike the Western biomedical model that focuses primarily on physical structures, the Eastern energetic paradigm offers a more holistic understanding of human existence—one that seamlessly integrates the physical, emotional, mental, and spiritual dimensions of our being. This chapter serves as both introduction and deep exploration of these concepts, providing both theoretical understanding and practical applications.

The Three Dantians: Power Centers of Energy

The term "Dantian" (丹田) literally translates as "elixir field" or "cinnabar field." In Chinese medicine and philosophical traditions such as Taoism, the Dantians are considered vital reservoirs of Qi (life energy) within the body. They function as both generators and storage centers for this essential life force. While many minor energy centers exist throughout the body, three primary Dantians serve as the main powerhouses of our energetic anatomy.

Lower Dantian (下丹田, Xia Dantian)

Located approximately two inches below the navel and about one-third of the way into the body, the Lower Dantian is often considered the most important of the three centers. In Japanese martial arts and meditation traditions, this region is known as "Hara," while yoga traditions refer to it as part of the Manipura or Svadhisthana chakra region.

The Lower Dantian serves as:

- The primary reservoir of Jing (essence) and Qi (vital energy)
- The foundation of physical power and stability
- The center of physical vitality and reproductive energy
- The "root" that connects us to the earth's energy

This center corresponds to our instinctual nature and relates to physical vitality, stamina, and our most basic survival functions. It is said that a person with strong Lower Dantian energy exhibits robust health, powerful physical presence, and remarkable endurance. Many qigong and meditation practices begin by focusing on this area to establish a solid energetic foundation before working with the higher centers.

Practical Focus: Lower Dantian Cultivation

To cultivate the Lower Dantian, practitioners often employ the following techniques:

- Deep abdominal breathing that expands and contracts the lower abdomen
- Standing meditation postures that direct attention and energy to this region
- Gentle rhythmic movements that massage and stimulate this area
- Visualization practices that imagine gathering light or energy in this center

Middle Dantian (中丹田, Zhong Dantian)

The Middle Dantian is located in the center of the chest at the level of the heart. This corresponds roughly to the heart chakra (Anahata) in yoga traditions. The Middle Dantian serves as the center for:

- Emotional processing and regulation
- Compassion and relationship with others
- The transformation of Qi into higher vibrational states
- The balance between self and other, inner and outer

This energy center mediates between the physical power of the Lower Dantian and the spiritual awareness of the Upper Dantian. It represents our capacity for emotional intelligence, empathy, and authentic connection with others. When the Middle Dantian is balanced and vibrant, we experience emotional stability, compassionate understanding, and harmonious relationships.

Practical Focus: Middle Dantian Cultivation

Practices for developing the Middle Dantian include:

- Heart-centered meditation that focuses on feelings of love and compassion
- Breath practices that expand and contract the chest region
- Sound healing that resonates with the chest cavity
- Visualization of a warm, radiant light emanating from the heart center

Upper Dantian (上丹田, Shang Dantian)

The Upper Dantian is located between the eyebrows and extends into the center of the brain. This corresponds to the "third eye" or Ajna chakra in yoga traditions. The Upper Dantian is associated with:

- Spiritual awareness and higher consciousness
- Intuition and inner wisdom
- Mental clarity and concentrated thought
- The refinement of Qi into Shen (spirit)

The Upper Dantian represents our capacity for transcendent awareness, insight, and connection to higher dimensions of consciousness. When this center is active and developed, one experiences enhanced intuition, mental clarity, and spiritual perception. Many advanced meditation practices focus on this center to cultivate heightened states of awareness.

Practical Focus: Upper Dantian Cultivation

To develop the Upper Dantian, practitioners employ:

- Silent meditation practices focusing attention at the point between the eyebrows
- Visualization of light or energy at this center
- Specific breathing techniques that direct energy upward to this region
- Sound vibrations that resonate with the head cavity

Integration of the Three Dantians

While each Dantian can be developed individually, true mastery comes from harmonizing and integrating all three centers. In many traditional practices, cultivation begins with the Lower Dantian to establish a solid foundation of vitality. As this foundation stabilizes, attention shifts to the Middle Dantian to refine emotional intelligence and harmonize relationships. Finally, focus moves to the Upper Dantian to develop spiritual awareness.

The ultimate goal is to establish a smooth flow of energy between all three centers, creating what is sometimes called the "small circulation" or "microcosmic orbit." This circulation allows energy to flow in a continuous loop from the Lower Dantian up the spine to the Upper Dantian and then down the front of the body back to the Lower Dantian, integrating all aspects of our being.

Meridians, Channels, and Energetic Anatomy

The Dantians serve as major energy reservoirs, but they are connected and empowered by an intricate network of energy pathways known as meridians or channels. This system forms the foundation of acupuncture, acupressure, and many energy cultivation practices.

The Meridian System Overview

In traditional Chinese medicine, the primary meridian system consists of 12 regular meridians and 8 extraordinary vessels. The regular meridians are bilateral (they appear on both sides of the body) and are associated with specific organs and functions. The extraordinary vessels act as reservoirs and regulators of energy throughout the system.

The 12 regular meridians include:

1. Lung Meridian
2. Large Intestine Meridian
3. Stomach Meridian
4. Spleen Meridian
5. Heart Meridian
6. Small Intestine Meridian
7. Bladder Meridian
8. Kidney Meridian
9. Pericardium Meridian
10. Triple Warmer Meridian (San Jiao)
11. Gallbladder Meridian
12. Liver Meridian

The 8 extraordinary vessels include:

1. Du Mai (Governing Vessel)
2. Ren Mai (Conception Vessel)
3. Chong Mai (Penetrating Vessel)
4. Dai Mai (Girdle Vessel)
5. Yang Qiao Mai (Yang Heel Vessel)
6. Yin Qiao Mai (Yin Heel Vessel)
7. Yang Wei Mai (Yang Linking Vessel)
8. Yin Wei Mai (Yin Linking Vessel)

Of these, the Du Mai and Ren Mai are particularly significant for energy cultivation practices as they form the primary pathways of the "microcosmic orbit" mentioned earlier.

Meridian Functions and Significance

Meridians serve several crucial functions in the energetic body:

1. **Energy Transportation**: They act as conduits for the flow of Qi throughout the body, nourishing tissues and supporting physiological functions.
2. **Information Transmission**: Meridians carry bioelectrical information that helps coordinate and regulate bodily functions.
3. **Homeostatic Regulation**: The meridian system plays a role in maintaining balance between yin and yang energies and among the five elements.
4. **Mind-Body Connection**: Meridians create bridges between physical organs and emotional/mental states.
5. **Spiritual Cultivation**: Certain meridians, particularly the extraordinary vessels, facilitate spiritual development and higher states of consciousness.

The meridians do not exist in isolation but form an integrated network throughout the body. Each meridian is connected to others at specific junction points, creating a web of energy that encompasses every aspect of our being.

Exploring Key Meridians for Energetic Development

While all meridians play important roles in health and well-being, certain pathways are particularly significant for energy cultivation practices:

The Governor Vessel (Du Mai): Running from the perineum up the spine to the top of the head and ending at the upper lip, this channel governs all yang energies in the body. It is associated with the nervous system and plays a crucial role in spiritual development.

The Conception Vessel (Ren Mai): Beginning at the perineum and traveling up the front midline of the body to the lower lip, this channel governs all yin energies and nourishes the internal organs.

The Penetrating Vessel (Chong Mai): Often called the "sea of blood," this vessel influences reproductive and ancestral energies and helps regulate the other meridians.

The Belt Channel (Dai Mai): The only horizontal meridian, it circles the waist like a belt and helps coordinate upper and lower energies in the body.

The Kidney Meridian: Beyond its association with the physical kidneys, this meridian stores our deepest essence (Jing) and governs development, reproduction, and longevity.

Understanding how to work with these key channels can dramatically enhance practices aimed at developing the three Dantians and integrating body, mind, and spirit.

Practical Applications: Working with the Meridian System

There are numerous ways to influence and balance the meridian system:

1. **Acupuncture and Acupressure**: Stimulating specific points along the meridians to regulate energy flow.
2. **Qigong and Tai Chi**: Movement practices that consciously direct energy through the meridians.
3. **Meridian Stretching**: Specific stretches designed to open and balance particular meridians.
4. **Self-Massage**: Techniques like self-acupressure or gua sha that stimulate meridian pathways.
5. **Visualization**: Mental practices that trace the path of energy through specific meridians.
6. **Sound Healing**: Using specific tones and vibrations that resonate with different meridians.

By working consciously with the meridian system, we can enhance the flow of energy to and between the three Dantians, creating greater harmony and integration throughout our entire being.

The Body-Mind-Spirit Relationship

The three Dantians and the meridian system provide the energetic infrastructure for the integration of body, mind, and spirit. Unlike the Western tendency to compartmentalize these aspects of our being, Eastern traditions recognize them as different dimensions of a unified whole.

The Triune Nature of Human Experience

In traditional Eastern paradigms, humans are understood to be composed of three treasures:

- **Jing** (精): The physical essence or substance, associated with the Lower Dantian
- **Qi** (气): The vital energy or life force, particularly associated with the Middle Dantian
- **Shen** (神): The spirit or consciousness, associated with the Upper Dantian

These three treasures correspond to body, energy/emotions, and mind/spirit respectively. They exist in a continuous spectrum, with each capable of transforming into the others through various alchemical practices.

The Body as Foundation

The physical body serves as the vessel for our life journey and the foundation for all energetic and spiritual development. Rather than viewing the body as separate from or inferior to the spirit, Eastern traditions honor the body as sacred and essential to spiritual cultivation.

Key principles regarding the body include:

- The body is the temple of the spirit and should be treated with reverence
- Physical health creates the foundation for emotional and spiritual well-being
- Bodily sensations provide important information about energy states
- The body stores memories and emotional patterns that affect consciousness
- Physical practices can directly influence mental and spiritual states

Practices that honor and develop the body include:

- Mindful movement practices like qigong and tai chi
- Proper nutrition according to energetic principles
- Adequate rest and sleep for restoration
- Contact with nature to ground and replenish

- Physical awareness practices to develop body intelligence

The Mind as Bridge

The mind functions as the bridge between physical and spiritual dimensions of experience. It both interprets physical sensations and receives spiritual insights. The Eastern understanding of mind encompasses both cognitive functions and emotional intelligence.

Important aspects of mind include:

- The distinction between "small mind" (ego/analytical thinking) and "big mind" (intuitive awareness)
- The recognition that thoughts directly influence energy flow and physical health
- The understanding that emotions are energetic states with physical correlates
- The practice of mental discipline as essential for spiritual development
- The cultivation of specific mind states that facilitate energy development

Practices for developing the mind include:

- Meditation to cultivate present-moment awareness
- Mindfulness of thoughts and emotions
- Visualization techniques to direct energy
- Study of wisdom teachings and contemplation
- Development of focused concentration

The Spirit as Guiding Light

Spirit represents the most subtle and transcendent aspect of our being. It encompasses our connection to universal consciousness, our deepest values and purpose, and our capacity for unconditional love and compassion.

Key aspects of spirit include:

- Our inherent connection to the universe and all beings
- The unique qualities of our individual soul or higher self
- Our capacity for transcendent states of consciousness
- Our ability to experience non-dual awareness
- Our innate drive toward growth, meaning, and purpose

Practices for spiritual cultivation include:

- Meditation on the nature of consciousness itself
- Cultivation of compassion and loving-kindness
- Service to others as an expression of spiritual realization
- Surrender to and trust in the greater wisdom of life
- Contemplation of existential questions about meaning and purpose

Integration: The Whole Being Path

The ultimate aim of working with the three Dantians and meridian system is to create harmony and integration among body, mind, and spirit. This integration happens through the conscious cultivation of energy and awareness.

When the three Dantians are balanced and connected through the meridian system:

- Physical health and vitality are enhanced (Lower Dantian)
- Emotional intelligence and heart-centered awareness flourish (Middle Dantian)
- Mental clarity and spiritual perception deepen (Upper Dantian)
- Energy flows smoothly throughout the entire system
- Body, mind, and spirit function as an integrated whole

This state of integration manifests as:

- Physical resilience and vitality
- Emotional balance and appropriate responsiveness
- Mental clarity and creativity
- Intuitive wisdom and insight
- Harmonious relationships with others
- Connection to purpose and meaning
- Present-moment awareness and joy

Practical Integration: A Daily Practice

To conclude this chapter, I offer a simple daily practice to help integrate the three Dantians and harmonize body, mind, and spirit:

1. **Begin with grounding (5 minutes)**:
   - Stand with feet shoulder-width apart, knees slightly bent
   - Feel your connection to the earth beneath you

- Breathe deeply into the Lower Dantian, imagining roots extending from your feet into the earth
- Gently rock or sway to release tension
2. **Activate the meridians (5-10 minutes)**:
   - Begin gentle tapping or patting along the major meridian pathways
   - Start at the crown of the head and work down the Governing Vessel
   - Continue along the inside and outside of the arms and legs
   - Finish by tapping up the Conception Vessel from pubic bone to chin
   - Feel the energy awakening throughout your body
3. **Three Dantian meditation (10-15 minutes)**:
   - Sit comfortably with a straight spine
   - Begin by focusing attention on the Lower Dantian, feeling warmth and vitality gather there (3-5 minutes)
   - Gradually shift awareness to the Middle Dantian, feeling a sense of openness and compassion (3-5 minutes)
   - Finally, bring attention to the Upper Dantian, experiencing clarity and spacious awareness (3-5 minutes)
   - Allow energy to circulate between all three centers, following the natural flow
4. **Integration and reflection (5 minutes)**:
   - Bring awareness to your entire being as an integrated whole
   - Notice how physical sensations, emotions, thoughts, and spiritual awareness are all aspects of your one experience
   - Reflect on how you might carry this integrated awareness into your day

This simple practice, performed regularly, can progressively transform your experience of body, mind, and spirit from seemingly separate domains into a harmonious whole.

The three Dantians, the meridian system, and the body-mind-spirit relationship offer a profound framework for understanding human experience beyond the limitations of mechanistic thinking. This energetic anatomy provides both a theoretical model and practical pathways for development and integration.

As you continue to explore these concepts through study and practice, remember that this knowledge was developed not merely as intellectual understanding but as lived experience to be validated through your own journey. The true test of these teachings lies not in their philosophical elegance but in their practical efficacy to transform your life.

May your exploration of these ancient wisdom traditions bring greater harmony, vitality, and awareness to every dimension of your being.

Here's your meditation rewritten as an easy-to-understand, **step-by-step guided exercise**, with a calm, gentle tone and clear instructions for each stage:

Qi Flow Exercise for Balancing Your Meridians

This exercise helps you clear blockages and restore the smooth flow of qi through your body's meridians.

Step 1: Get Comfortable & Set Your Intention

1. **Find a quiet place.** Sit with your spine straight or lie down, comfortably supported.
2. **Rest your hands** on your lap or by your sides.
3. **Take 3 deep breaths:**
   - Inhale slowly through your nose…
   - Exhale gently through your mouth…
   - With each breath, feel your body soften and relax.
4. **Silently say:**
   "I welcome the free, balanced flow of qi throughout my body. I release all blockages and embrace vibrant energy."

Step 2: Connect with Your Qi

1. **Visualize your breath** drawing in healing, luminous energy with each inhale.
2. **As you exhale,** imagine heavy or stagnant energy leaving your body.
3. **Picture your qi** as a glowing, radiant light inside you—gentle, warm, and alive.
4. **Feel it flowing** freely, ready to be guided along your energy pathways.

Step 3: Guide the Qi Through Your Meridians

a. Upper Body: Breath and Heart

1. **Lung and Large Intestine Meridians**
   - Focus on your chest.
   - Imagine qi filling your lungs with light.
   - See it flowing from your lungs along the meridians down to your fingers.
   - Let any blockages dissolve into light.
2. **Heart and Pericardium Meridians**
   - Shift awareness to your heart.
   - Visualize warm, radiant energy entering your heart center.
   - Let it pulse outward through your chest along the pericardium meridian.
   - Feel your heart open and soften.

b. Arms and Digestive Area

3. **Spleen and Stomach Meridians**
   - Bring your focus to your abdomen.
   - See the qi moving from your heart into your belly.
   - Let it travel down the spleen and stomach meridians.
   - Visualize it warming and clearing your digestive area.
4. **Small Intestine and Triple Burner Meridians**
   - Now, focus on your arms.
   - Watch the qi rise and flow through the small intestine and triple burner meridians.
   - Let it reach all the way to your fingertips.
   - With each breath out, see blockages melt away like morning mist.

Lower Body: Grounding and Flow

5. **Kidney and Bladder Meridians**
   - Focus on your lower back and hips.
   - Visualize qi grounding into your kidneys like fresh water flowing down.

- o Let it run down your legs through the bladder meridian.
- o Feel knots or tension dissolving in a clear, refreshing current.

6. **Liver and Gallbladder Meridians**
   - o Turn your attention to the sides of your body.
   - o Imagine qi circulating along your liver and gallbladder meridians.
   - o See it cleansing and re-energizing every cell along its path.

Step 4: Deepen and Harmonize

1. **Sense the energy** now flowing smoothly through all your meridians.
2. **Visualize your body glowing** brighter with each breath—your energy system unified and radiant.
3. **If you feel tension or darkness**, gently breathe into that area.
   - o With each exhale, imagine the light washing the tension away.
   - o See clarity and brightness take its place.

Step 5: Complete and Return

1. **Rest in the sensation** of balance and openness.
2. **Feel your whole body alive** with light and harmony.
3. **Begin to return slowly:**
   - o Notice your breath again.
   - o Feel the surface beneath you.
   - o Wiggle your fingers and toes gently.
4. **Take one final deep breath.**
   - o As you exhale, softly open your eyes.

Closing Reflection

Take a quiet moment to feel gratitude for your practice.
Know that this smooth, vibrant flow of qi is always within you.
You can return to this space anytime to recharge, balance, and reconnect.

Below is a **meditation audio script** version of the *Qi Flow Meridians Exercise*, designed to be spoken in a calm, steady, and soothing voice, with natural pauses between lines to allow the listener to follow along with ease. You can read this to yourself or record it.

Qi Flow Meridians Meditation

Welcome.
This is a guided meditation to balance the flow of qi—your life force energy—through your meridians.

Let's begin by finding a quiet, comfortable space.
You may sit upright with your spine gently aligned…
Or lie down in a supported, relaxed position.
Let your hands rest softly…
On your lap or by your sides.

Now… take a slow, deep breath in through your nose…
And exhale gently through your mouth.

Again…
Inhale…
Exhale…
One more time…
Let go of any tension.
Let your body begin to soften.
Let your mind begin to quiet.

Now, silently say to yourself:
"I welcome the free, balanced flow of qi throughout my body. I release all blockages and embrace vibrant energy."

Let this intention guide your practice.

Bring your awareness to your breath.
With every inhale… imagine you're drawing in luminous, healing energy.
With every exhale… release any heaviness, tension, or stagnant energy.

Now visualize a radiant, gentle light filling your body.
This is your qi…
Warm, alive, flowing.

Let's begin to guide this qi through the meridians of your body.

Focus on your chest.
As you breathe, see the light entering your lungs…
Expanding with each inhale…
Now visualize it flowing through the lung meridians…
Down your arms…
To your fingertips.

Let any heaviness or blockages melt away in the flow of light.

Now, bring your focus to your heart.
Feel the qi nourishing your heart center…
Warmth…
Compassion…
Let it gently pulse through your chest…
Flowing through the pericardium meridian.

Feel your heart expand and soften.

Now move your attention to your belly.
Let the qi move downward from your heart…
Into your abdomen.
Visualize it traveling through the spleen and stomach meridians…
Warming…
Cleansing…
Bringing balance.

Now guide the qi up your arms…
Feel it rising through the small intestine and triple burner meridians…
All the way to your fingertips.
With every breath, feel the energy clearing…
Lightening…
Flowing freely.

Now shift your awareness to your lower back and hips.
Let the energy ground into your kidneys…
Calm…
Stable…
Visualize it flowing down through the kidney meridian…
Then the bladder meridian…
Washing through your legs…
All the way to your feet.

Feel knots of tension dissolve.
Feel clarity and refreshment.

Now bring attention to the sides of your body.
Visualize qi flowing through the liver and gallbladder meridians.
Cleansing…
Balancing…
Energizing each cell it touches.

Breathe slowly and deeply.
Let the qi now move freely through all the pathways.
A continuous circuit…
A glowing flow of light.
Let it harmonize your whole being.

If you sense any resistance, any darkness…
Gently breathe into it.
Exhale and release.
Let the light dissolve and transform it.
Feel the qi becoming smooth, bright, and unified.

Now… simply rest in this radiant flow.
Enjoy the feeling of openness…
Lightness…
And balance.

Begin to bring your awareness back to your breath…
The gentle rise and fall of your chest…
The sensations in your body…
The support beneath you…
And the space around you.

Take one final, deep breath in…
And as you exhale…
Gently open your eyes.

Take a moment now…
To appreciate how you feel.
Know that this state of balance is always available to you.
With regular practice, you can keep your qi flowing freely…
Nurturing your health, clarity, and well-being.

Thank you for joining this meditation.
May your qi flow with ease…
Bringing harmony to every part of your life.

The Foundation of Internal Energy Development

Aligning Posture: Zhan Zhuang Basics

Zhan Zhuang, or "standing like a tree," is a foundational practice in many Chinese internal martial arts and qigong systems. This deceptively simple practice of standing in specific postures builds tremendous internal strength, stability, and energy awareness.

At its core, Zhan Zhuang teaches proper structural alignment—allowing gravity to flow through the body with minimal muscular effort. When the body is properly aligned, energy (qi) flows more efficiently, muscles can relax while maintaining structure, and the practitioner develops a profound sense of rootedness.

The practice involves maintaining static postures for gradually increasing periods of time. These postures appear simple but require precise alignment and relaxed attention to detail. Through consistent practice, the body develops what the Chinese call "sung"—a state of alert relaxation where unnecessary tension dissolves while necessary structure remains.

Key elements of proper alignment include:

- Feet parallel and shoulder-width apart
- Knees slightly bent, never locked
- Pelvis slightly tucked, avoiding excessive anterior or posterior tilt
- Spine elongated but maintaining natural curves
- Shoulders relaxed and slightly rounded
- Arms positioned as if gently embracing a large tree
- Head balanced as if suspended from above

Exercises for Aligning Posture

Wuji is the foundational standing posture used in Nei Gong and Qigong. It represents a state of neutrality, balance, and readiness—physically and energetically.

How to Practice Wuji Posture:

1. **Stand with feet shoulder-width apart**
   Keep your feet flat and parallel, with toes pointing straight ahead.
2. **Slightly bend your knees**
   Avoid locking the knees; let them stay soft and relaxed.
3. **Tuck your pelvis slightly**
   Gently roll your hips under to straighten the lower back. Imagine your tailbone dropping toward the ground.
4. **Align the spine**
   Imagine your head is suspended from above by a string. Let the crown lift slightly while the chin tucks just a bit to elongate the neck.
5. **Relax your shoulders and arms**
   Let your arms hang loosely by your sides or form a gentle circle in front of the lower abdomen (like holding a beach ball).
6. **Soften your gaze or close your eyes**
   Bring your attention inward, resting lightly in your breath and body.
7. **Breathe slowly and deeply**
   Let each breath flow down into your Lower Dantian (below the navel), expanding naturally with each inhale.

Exercise 1: Finding Structural Alignment (Hugging a Tree)

1. Stand with feet parallel, shoulder-width apart
2. Slightly bend your knees, feeling weight sink into your feet
3. Gently tuck your tailbone, allowing your lower back to lengthen
4. Imagine your spine growing taller, creating space between vertebrae
5. Relax your shoulders down and slightly forward
6. Hold your arms as if embracing a tree, elbows pointing down
7. Tuck your chin slightly, imagining a thread pulling the crown of your head upward
8. Hold for 2 minutes initially, gradually increasing time

9. Focus on releasing unnecessary tension while maintaining the structure

Exercise 2: Scanning for Tension

1. Assume the basic standing posture from Exercise 1
2. Close your eyes and mentally scan your body from feet to head
3. When you notice tension, consciously relax that area without losing structure
4. Pay special attention to common tension areas: jaw, shoulders, lower back
5. Continue cycling through the body for 5-10 minutes
6. Each time you exhale, imagine releasing another layer of unnecessary tension

Exercise 3: Micro-Adjustments

1. Stand in the basic posture with a wall behind you
2. Have your heels, buttocks, upper back, and head lightly touching the wall
3. Step away from the wall while maintaining this alignment
4. Make tiny adjustments until you feel "stacked" with minimal effort
5. Test your alignment by having a partner gently push on your sternum
6. If you easily lose balance, refine your alignment and try again
7. Practice daily for 5 minutes, gradually increasing to 15-20 minutes

Breathing Practices for Grounding

Breath is the bridge between the conscious and unconscious mind, between voluntary and involuntary function. In internal arts, specific breathing methods create a profound sense of groundedness—connecting the practitioner to both the earth below and the heavens above.

Proper breathing practices stimulate the vagus nerve, activating the parasympathetic nervous system and creating a calm, centered state. When combined with aligned posture, these breathing techniques enhance stability, focus, and energy circulation throughout the body.

The most fundamental breathing approach in internal arts is abdominal or "dan tian" breathing. This method of breathing into the lower abdomen encourages a deeper connection to one's center of gravity, promoting stability and energy storage.

Exercise 1: Abdominal Breathing Awareness

1. Sit comfortably with your spine erect or lie on your back
2. Place one hand on your chest and one on your lower abdomen
3. Breathe normally for 1 minute, observing your current pattern
4. Gradually shift your breath so that your lower hand rises with each inhale
5. Keep your chest relatively still, allowing the abdomen to expand
6. Make each breath smooth, continuous, and without strain
7. Practice for 5 minutes, gradually increasing to 15 minutes
8. Eventually transition to practicing while standing in Zhan Zhuang

Exercise 2: Rooting Breath

1. Stand in the basic Zhan Zhuang posture
2. As you inhale, imagine drawing energy up from the earth through your feet
3. As you exhale, visualize this energy flowing down to your lower dan tian (below navel)
4. With each breath cycle, feel an increasing sense of heaviness and connection to the ground
5. Keep your breathing quiet, smooth, and unhurried
6. Continue for 10-15 minutes, maintaining structural alignment
7. Notice how your stability increases as your breathing deepens

Exercise 3: Three-Part Breathing

1. Begin in standing or seated position with good alignment
2. Inhale first into your lower abdomen, feeling it expand
3. Continue the same inhale, allowing it to fill the middle torso
4. Complete the inhale by allowing the upper chest to expand slightly
5. Exhale in reverse order: upper chest, middle torso, lower abdomen
6. Make each breath phase seamless, without pauses
7. Practice for 10 cycles, then rest and observe the effects
8. Gradually increase to 36 breath cycles
9. Apply this breathing pattern while practicing Zhan Zhuang

Ting Jing, or "listening energy," is the refined sensitivity that allows a practitioner to perceive subtle energetic changes within themselves and others. This skill forms the foundation of the highest levels of internal martial arts and energy cultivation.

At its essence, Ting Jing requires turning awareness inward, developing an increasingly refined perception of internal states. This includes awareness of minute muscular tensions, subtle energy movements, emotional states, and even the quality of one's thoughts.

In martial applications, this sensitivity extends outward, allowing the practitioner to "listen" to an opponent's intentions before they manifest physically. In healing arts, it enables precise diagnosis and treatment. In daily life, it creates a heightened awareness that enriches every experience.

Developing Ting Jing requires patient, consistent practice with a quiet, receptive mind. The practitioner learns to distinguish between different qualities of sensation, developing what some traditions call "educated touch."

Exercises for Developing Inner Listening

Exercise 1: Single-Point Awareness

1. Sit or stand in a comfortable, aligned position
2. Bring your full attention to a single point in your body (tip of index finger recommended for beginners)
3. Notice all sensations at this point: temperature, pressure, tingling, pulsing
4. When your mind wanders, gently return to the sensations at this point
5. Practice for 5 minutes initially, gradually increasing to 15
6. Over time, choose increasingly subtle points to focus on
7. Eventually practice while in Zhan Zhuang posture

Exercise 2: Energy Pathways Awareness

1. Stand in the basic Zhan Zhuang posture
2. Focus your attention on your right palm
3. Without moving, imagine energy flowing from your palm to your wrist
4. Continue tracing this pathway up the arm to the shoulder
5. Then follow the energy across the upper back to the left shoulder
6. Continue down the left arm to the left palm

7. Reverse the direction, following from left palm back to right
8. Practice for 10 minutes, keeping your breathing natural
9. Notice any sensations that arise along this pathway

Exercise 3: Whole-Body Listening

1. Begin in a comfortably aligned standing position
2. Close your eyes and expand your awareness to include your entire body
3. Rather than focusing on any particular area, maintain a diffuse awareness
4. Notice the subtle pulsations, vibrations, and energy movements throughout
5. If you notice yourself focusing too intently on one area, gently expand awareness again
6. Practice maintaining this whole-body awareness for 10-20 minutes
7. Eventually integrate this awareness with the aligned posture and breathing practices
8. Practice "listening" to your body during daily activities, not just formal practice

Integration: The Three Pillars Working Together

These three practices—aligned posture, grounding breath, and inner listening—form the foundation of all advanced internal energy work. When practiced together, they create a powerful synergy that accelerates development.

Integration Exercise: The Three Harmonies

1. Begin with structural alignment, establishing the basic Zhan Zhuang posture
2. Once aligned, introduce abdominal breathing, feeling each breath ground you further
3. As your breathing stabilizes, expand your awareness to include the entire body
4. Notice how alignment affects your breathing and energy awareness
5. Notice how breathing affects your structural stability and sensitivity
6. Notice how inner listening reveals areas of tension that affect alignment and breath
7. Continue this integrated practice for 20-30 minutes
8. After practice, spend 5 minutes journaling your observations
9. Make this integrated practice a daily cornerstone of your training

Through consistent practice of these three foundational skills, the practitioner develops what the classics call "whole-body awareness" and "whole-body power."

These qualities provide the necessary foundation for all advanced internal energy cultivation and application.

Journal Reflection

Contemplate: *"What is my intention for inner cultivation?"*

Take a few quiet moments before practice. Write honestly and clearly.

- Why have you chosen this path?
- What do you wish to transform or awaken within yourself?
- What qualities—physical, emotional, or spiritual—do you want to embody more fully?

Your Reflection:

_____
_____
_____
_____
_____
_____

Review Exercise: Align and Breathe (10 Minutes)

This simple exercise harmonizes your structure and calming the internal system.

Instructions:

1. Stand in Wuji posture or sit comfortably.
2. Align head, spine, and pelvis. Soften knees if standing.
3. Allow your shoulders to drop and your belly to relax.
4. Breathe slowly through the nose into your Lower Dantian (about 2 inches below the navel).
5. Let each exhale release tension.
6. Stay present with your breath and body for 10 minutes.

Optional Tip: Set a timer and begin with just 5 minutes if needed.

Afterward, reflect below:

- What sensations did you notice?
- Did your mind wander? What helped you return to the present?

Notes:

_____

_____

_____

Body Scan & Tension Awareness Tracker

This scan helps you identify where you hold unconscious tension and begin the process of releasing it.

Instructions:

- Either standing or sitting, close your eyes and slowly scan from head to toe.
- At each region, observe any sensation: tension, tightness, warmth, numbness, etc.
- No need to fix or judge—just notice.

Body Region	Sensation or Tension Detected
Head & Face	
Neck & Shoulders	
Chest & Heart	
Abdomen & Lower Back	
Hips & Pelvis	
Legs & Knees	
Feet	

Optional: *Where do I habitually store stress?*

PART II: Nei Gong – Refining Jing into Qi

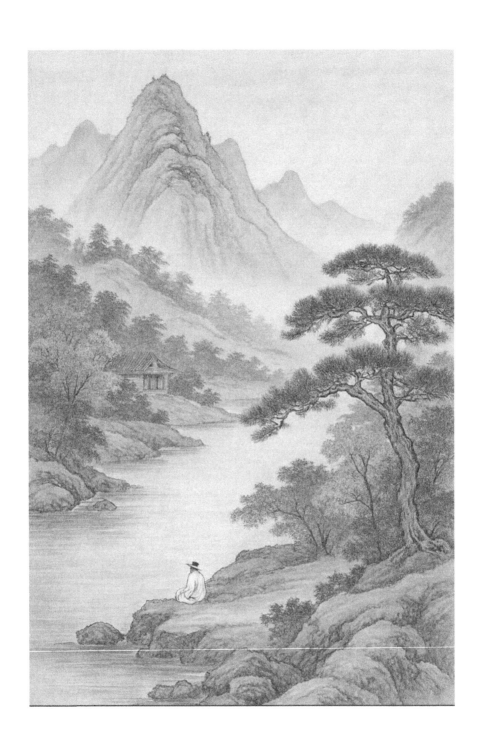

Chapter 4: Lower Dantian Power

The lower dantian (下丹田), located in the lower abdomen approximately three finger widths below the navel and two finger widths inward, serves as the body's primary energy reservoir in qigong and internal martial arts practices. Often described as a cauldron or furnace for qi cultivation, the lower dantian functions as both generator and storage facility for vital energy.

In this chapter, we explore methods to build, fill, and expand this crucial energy center. By developing your lower dantian, you establish the foundation for advanced energy work, increased vitality, and powerful internal expression in martial applications.

Understanding the Lower Dantian

Before diving into practices, let's establish a clear understanding of the lower dantian's role in energy cultivation:

1. **Foundation of Energy**: The lower dantian serves as the root of all energy development in the body.
2. **Storage Capacity**: Like a battery or reservoir, it holds accumulated qi for later use.
3. **Transformation Center**: Raw energy is refined here before circulating throughout the body.
4. **Physical Strength Connection**: A developed lower dantian improves core stability and power generation.

Traditional Taoist texts describe the lower dantian as "the root of the tree of life" and "the ocean of qi." When properly developed, it becomes a tangible sensation in your practice—a center of warmth, fullness, and vibrant energy.

Building and Filling the Energy Reservoir

The process of developing the lower dantian involves consistent practice of specific techniques designed to draw energy into this center and expand its capacity. Think of this as both constructing a vessel and filling it simultaneously.

Exercise 1: Dantian Awareness Meditation

Purpose: To establish direct awareness of the lower dantian region.

Practice:

1. Sit comfortably in a chair or cross-legged on the floor with your spine erect.
2. Place both palms over your lower abdomen, with your thumbs at navel level and your fingertips pointing toward your pubic bone.
3. Close your eyes and take several natural breaths.
4. Direct your attention to the space beneath your palms, approximately two inches inside your body.
5. Mentally create a small sphere of energy in this location—picture it as a pearl of light or a warm sensation.
6. Maintain awareness of this point for 5-10 minutes without straining.
7. When your mind wanders, gently return focus to the dantian.

Progression:

- Begin with 5-minute sessions, gradually extending to 15-20 minutes.
- As your sensitivity develops, practice without hand placement, maintaining mental focus alone.
- Note any sensations that develop: warmth, pulsing, expansion, or fullness.

Exercise 2: Dantian Breathing

Purpose: To direct breath energy into the lower dantian.

Practice:

1. Stand in a relaxed position with feet shoulder-width apart, knees slightly bent.
2. Place one palm over your lower dantian.
3. Inhale slowly through your nose, visualizing energy entering through either the nose or the crown of your head.
4. Guide this energy down to your lower dantian.
5. As you exhale through your nose, imagine the energy condensing and being stored in your dantian.
6. With each breath cycle, perceive the dantian growing warmer and more substantial.
7. Continue for 5-10 minutes.

Progression:

- Begin with 5 minutes daily, gradually increasing to 15-20 minutes.
- As you progress, sense the dantian becoming more defined with each practice session.
- Eventually, maintain dantian awareness throughout normal daily activities.

Exercise 3: Energy Cycling

Purpose: To circulate energy through the body, returning it to the dantian for storage.

Practice:

1. Begin in a seated or standing position with eyes closed.
2. Establish awareness of your lower dantian through several focused breaths.
3. On inhalation, visualize energy rising from the dantian up the spine to the crown.
4. On exhalation, guide the energy down the front of the body (conception vessel) back to the dantian.
5. Complete 9, 18, or 36 cycles, maintaining smooth, continuous circulation.

Progression:

- Start with slow, deliberate cycles focusing on clear visualization.
- Gradually increase speed while maintaining quality of awareness.
- Eventually, the energy should flow in a continuous circuit without rigid attachment to breath.

Diaphragmatic Breathing

Proper breathing forms the cornerstone of dantian development. Diaphragmatic breathing, also called abdominal or belly breathing, directly engages and strengthens the lower dantian while maximizing oxygen intake and energy conversion.

Understanding Diaphragmatic Breathing

The diaphragm is a dome-shaped muscle separating the chest and abdominal cavities. When you inhale correctly, the diaphragm contracts and flattens, creating negative pressure that draws air into the lungs while pushing the abdomen outward.

During exhalation, the diaphragm relaxes, returning to its dome shape, pressing against the lungs and expelling air.

This natural breathing mechanism:

- Massages internal organs
- Increases oxygen exchange efficiency
- Directly stimulates the lower dantian
- Activates the parasympathetic nervous system (relaxation response)
- Improves lymphatic circulation

Exercise 4: Fundamental Diaphragmatic Breathing

Purpose: To establish proper diaphragmatic breathing mechanics.

Practice:

1. Lie on your back with knees bent, feet flat on the floor.
2. Place one hand on your chest and the other on your abdomen just below the ribcage.
3. Breathe slowly through your nose, directing the breath deep into your lungs.
4. The hand on your abdomen should rise substantially, while the hand on your chest remains relatively still.
5. Exhale slowly through slightly pursed lips, feeling your abdominal hand lower.
6. Focus on making each breath smooth, deep, and relaxed, without forcing or straining.
7. Practice for 5 minutes initially, gradually increasing duration.

Progression:

- Once comfortable lying down, practice sitting upright.
- Progress to standing practice.
- Eventually integrate this breathing pattern into daily activities and other exercises.

Exercise 5: Reverse Breathing

Purpose: To develop advanced control of the dantian and internal pressure.

Note: Master basic diaphragmatic breathing before attempting reverse breathing.

Practice:

1. Stand in a relaxed position with feet shoulder-width apart.
2. Place hands lightly over the lower dantian.
3. Inhale slowly through the nose, gently contracting the lower abdomen (drawing the navel slightly inward).
4. Simultaneously, expand the lower back and sides of the waist.
5. Exhale through the nose, allowing the abdomen to expand outward while the lower back contracts slightly.
6. Maintain relaxation throughout, avoiding excessive tension.
7. Practice for 3-5 minutes initially.

Progression:

- Begin with just 3-5 minutes of practice, as reverse breathing can be taxing initially.
- Gradually extend duration as comfort increases.
- Eventually, learn to switch between normal and reverse breathing based on specific applications.

Exercise 6: Dantian Breathing Sphere

Purpose: To coordinate breath with dantian energy expansion and contraction.

Practice:

1. Stand in a comfortable stance with knees slightly bent.
2. Place hands in front of the lower dantian, palms facing each other about 8 inches apart.
3. As you inhale, slowly move your hands apart, imagining the dantian expanding like a balloon.
4. Simultaneously, feel expansion in your lower abdomen and lower back.
5. As you exhale, gradually bring your hands closer (but not touching), visualizing the dantian condensing and becoming more concentrated.
6. Repeat for 5-10 minutes, maintaining relaxed attention.

Progression:

- Begin with small, subtle movements.
- Gradually increase the range of expansion and contraction.

- Eventually, perform without hand movements, using only internal awareness.

Dantian Focusing and Expansion

Once basic awareness and breathing techniques are established, we can proceed to more focused dantian development exercises. These practices concentrate qi in the lower dantian and gradually expand its capacity and power.

Exercise 7: Dantian Condensation

Purpose: To concentrate energy in the lower dantian.

Practice:

1. Stand in a relaxed position with feet shoulder-width apart, knees slightly bent.
2. Place your palms over the lower dantian.
3. Close your eyes and establish dantian awareness through several breaths.
4. Visualize drawing energy from all parts of your body—limbs, head, torso— toward your dantian.
5. With each exhalation, imagine this energy becoming more concentrated and refined.
6. Sense the dantian becoming warmer, denser, and more tangible.
7. Continue for 5-10 minutes.

Progression:

- Begin with short sessions focusing on clear sensation.
- Gradually extend duration as concentration improves.
- Eventually, practice condensing energy from the environment as well as from within your body.

Exercise 8: Dantian Expansion

Purpose: To increase the capacity and influence of the dantian.

Practice:

1. Begin with dantian condensation until you feel a clear sensation of concentrated energy.

2. Then, on inhalations, visualize the dantian expanding outward in all directions.
3. With each breath, allow the sphere of energy to grow larger—first filling your lower abdomen, then your entire torso.
4. Maintain the quality and integrity of the energy as it expands.
5. On exhalations, stabilize the expanded field without contracting it.
6. Continue for 5-10 minutes.

Progression:

- Start with modest expansion, focusing on maintaining clear sensation.
- Gradually increase the range of expansion with practice.
- Eventually, practice expanding the energy field to encompass your entire body and beyond.

Exercise 9: Dantian Pulsing

Purpose: To develop dynamic control of dantian energy.

Practice:

1. Stand or sit with attention focused on your lower dantian.
2. Establish a clear sensation of energy in this center.
3. Begin gentle, rhythmic expansion and contraction of the dantian—like a heart beating or a jellyfish pulsing.
4. Coordinate this pulsing with your breath initially (expand on inhale, contract on exhale).
5. As you progress, the pulsing can become independent of breathing rhythm.
6. Maintain for 3-5 minutes.

Progression:

- Begin with slow, subtle pulsations.
- Gradually increase the intensity and range of pulsation.
- Eventually, practice varying the rhythm and intensity, developing fine control.

Exercise 10: Dan-Zhong Connection

Purpose: To establish energy connection between lower and middle dantians.

Practice:

1. Sit or stand in a relaxed position.
2. Place one hand over your lower dantian and the other over your middle dantian (center of chest).
3. Focus attention on both centers simultaneously.
4. As you inhale, visualize energy rising from the lower dantian to the middle dantian.
5. As you exhale, visualize energy descending from the middle dantian back to the lower dantian.
6. After several minutes, sense a permanent energetic bridge between these centers.
7. Practice for 5-10 minutes.

Progression:

- Begin with clear focus on the distinct sensation of each center.
- Gradually refine awareness of the pathway connecting them.
- Eventually, establish instant connection between centers without deliberate visualization.

Integration Practices

The following exercises help integrate dantian power into movement and daily activities.

Exercise 11: Walking With Dantian Awareness

Purpose: To maintain dantian awareness during movement.

Practice:

1. Begin standing with clear dantian awareness.
2. Start walking slowly, maintaining constant awareness of your energy center.
3. Feel as though you are moving from the dantian rather than from the legs.
4. Sense how the dantian remains stable while the body moves around it.
5. Gradually increase walking speed while maintaining awareness.
6. Practice for 10-15 minutes.

Progression:

- Start with slow, mindful walking.
- Progress to normal walking speed.
- Eventually, maintain awareness during various activities: climbing stairs, reaching, bending, etc.

Purpose: To express physical movement from the dantian.

Practice:

1. Stand in a relaxed position with clear dantian awareness.
2. Begin simple arm movements—circles, pushing, pulling—initiating each movement from the dantian.
3. Feel energy flowing from the dantian through the waist, into the shoulders, and out through the arms.
4. Move slowly and mindfully, ensuring each action originates from your center.
5. Practice basic movements for 10-15 minutes.

Progression:

- Begin with simple arm movements.
- Progress to whole-body movements.
- Eventually, apply this awareness to martial forms or daily activities.

Common Challenges and Solutions

Challenge: Difficulty Sensing the Dantian

Solution:

- Use physical touch to establish location—place three fingers below navel.
- Try practicing after moderate exercise when body awareness is heightened.
- Use visualization of warmth, light, or a small dense ball in the correct location.
- Be patient; sensation develops gradually with consistent practice.

Challenge: Mind Wandering During Practice

Solution:

- Begin with shorter practice periods (3-5 minutes).
- Use counting to structure breathing (count each complete breath cycle).
- Return to the practice without self-judgment when you notice wandering.
- Consider using subtle background sounds (soft drone or natural sounds) to anchor attention.

Challenge: Tension or Discomfort During Practice

Solution:

- Reduce effort and practice with less intensity.
- Ensure proper posture without rigidity.
- Incorporate gentle movement before static practice.
- Never force sensations; allow them to develop naturally.

Signs of Progress

As you develop your lower dantian through consistent practice, you may experience some of these indicators of progress:

1. **Thermal Sensations**: Warmth, sometimes intense, in the lower abdomen.
2. **Energetic Awareness**: Clear perception of the dantian, even without focused attention.
3. **Expanded Breathing Capacity**: Deeper, more efficient breathing patterns.
4. **Improved Digestive Function**: Better appetite regulation and digestion.
5. **Enhanced Core Stability**: Improved balance and postural alignment.
6. **Increased Energy Levels**: Greater vitality and reduced fatigue.
7. **Emotional Stability**: Calmer responses to stressful situations.
8. **Intuitive Movement**: Physical actions naturally originate from the center.

Remember that progress varies greatly between individuals. Some may experience noticeable sensations within weeks, while others may practice for months before clear perceptions develop. The key is consistency rather than intensity.

The development of lower dantian power forms the foundation for all advanced energy work. Through the practices presented in this chapter, you have begun establishing both the awareness and capacity of this vital energy center.

Practice these exercises with patience and consistency. As Laozi reminds us in the Tao De Jing: "A journey of a thousand miles begins with a single step." Similarly, developing profound dantian power begins with simple, repeated attention to your energetic center.

In the next chapter, we will explore techniques for circulating this cultivated energy through the primary meridian pathways, further enhancing your internal development and laying the groundwork for practical applications.

Recommended Practice Schedule

Week 1-2: Foundation

- Dantian Awareness Meditation: 5 minutes, twice daily
- Fundamental Diaphragmatic Breathing: 5 minutes, twice daily
- Walking With Dantian Awareness: 5 minutes daily

Week 3-4: Development

- Dantian Breathing: 5 minutes, twice daily
- Energy Cycling: 9 cycles, once daily
- Dantian Condensation: 5 minutes, once daily
- Continue Walking With Dantian Awareness: 10 minutes daily

Week 5-6: Expansion

- Energy Cycling: 18 cycles, once daily
- Dantian Expansion: 5 minutes, once daily
- Dantian Pulsing: 3 minutes, once daily
- Dantian-Centered Movement: 5-10 minutes, once daily
- Integrate awareness into daily activities

Week 7-8: Integration

- Combine practices as intuition guides
- Minimum 30 minutes total daily practice
- Focus on quality of sensation rather than quantity of exercises
- Begin connecting with practices from previous chapters

Journal Reflection

Contemplate: "What is my current relationship with my lower dantian?"
Explore your initial awareness, expectations, and intentions around cultivating this energy center.

Your Reflection:

_____

————

Practice Log: Dantian Awareness & Breathing

Track your daily practice for the week. Note how long you practiced and any sensations or changes you noticed.

Date	Exercise Practiced	Duration (min)	Notes (sensations, awareness, focus)

Body Scan & Dantian Sensation Awareness

Use this space to map your internal sensations before and after Dantian practices. Note any warmth, pressure, expansion, or pulsing in specific areas.

Body Region	Before Practice	After Practice
Lower Abdomen / Dantian		
Lower Back		
Pelvic Floor		
Thighs / Hips		
Upper Abdomen		
Breathing Depth (before and after)		

"Energy flows where attention goes." — Ancient Taoist saying

The human body is a complex network of energy channels, known in various traditions as meridians, nadis, or in Taoist practice, as the "mai." These channels transport life force energy (qi or chi) throughout our entire being, nourishing our physical body, emotional landscape, and spiritual essence.

When these channels are open and qi flows freely, we experience vibrant health, emotional balance, and spiritual clarity. When blockages occur—due to stress, poor posture, emotional suppression, or other factors—we may experience discomfort, disease, or a sense of disconnection from our true nature.

This chapter explores three fundamental practices for opening energy channels and cultivating harmonious qi flow:

1. **The Microcosmic Orbit**: The master circuit that connects all major energy centers
2. **Spinal Opening and Breath**: Techniques to release blockages along the central channel
3. **Energy Ball Between Hands Practice**: A method to sensitize your awareness to qi and build your capacity to direct it

These practices form the foundation of more advanced energy work. By mastering them, you create the conditions for deeper healing, spiritual insight, and the eventual awakening of latent potentials within your energetic system.

Let us begin this journey with patience and curiosity, remembering that energy work is both an art and a science—requiring both disciplined practice and intuitive exploration.

Part I: The Microcosmic Orbit

Understanding the Microcosmic Orbit

The Microcosmic Orbit, also known as the "Small Heavenly Circuit" (Xiao Zhou Tian), is the primary energy pathway in Taoist internal alchemy. It consists of two main channels:

1. **The Governing Vessel (Du Mai)**: Rising up the spine from the perineum to the crown and then to the upper palate
2. **The Conception Vessel (Ren Mai)**: Descending down the front of the body from the lower lip to the perineum

When these two channels connect, they form a complete circuit of energy that harmonizes yin and yang forces within the body. Regular practice of the Microcosmic Orbit is said to:

- Increase vitality and longevity
- Clear energy blockages
- Balance the nervous system
- Promote emotional stability
- Create the foundation for higher spiritual development

The Microcosmic Orbit naturally circulates to some degree in everyone, but conscious cultivation significantly enhances its benefits and prepares the body-mind system for more advanced energy practices.

Exercises for the Microcosmic Orbit

Exercise 1: Preparing the Path

Purpose: To familiarize yourself with the route of the Microcosmic Orbit before attempting to circulate energy through it.

Preparation:

- Find a quiet space where you won't be disturbed for at least 20 minutes
- Wear loose, comfortable clothing
- Sit in a comfortable position with your spine straight (on a chair or in a meditation posture)

Steps:

1. Place your hands comfortably on your lap or knees
2. Close your eyes and take 9 deep, slow breaths to center yourself
3. Bring your attention to your lower abdomen (lower dantian), about 1.5 inches below your navel and 2 inches inward
4. Imagine this area as a sphere of warm, golden light
5. From this starting point, mentally trace the following route:

- From the lower dantian down to the perineum (the Huiyin or "gate of life" point)
- Up the spine, passing through:
  - The sacrum
  - The lumbar region (lower back)
  - Between the kidneys
  - Between the shoulder blades
  - The base of the skull
  - The crown of the head (Baihui point)
- Down the front of the face, passing through:
  - The third eye point (between the eyebrows)
  - The tip of the nose
  - The upper lip
  - The lower lip
- Continue down the front center line of the body, passing through:
  - The throat
  - The center of the chest (heart center)
  - The solar plexus
  - Return to the lower dantian

6. Trace this route with your awareness 3 times, spending about 30 seconds at each major point
7. After completing the third round, rest your awareness in the lower dantian for 2-3 minutes
8. Gently rub your palms together until warm, then massage your face and smooth your energy field by brushing down your torso and limbs
9. Slowly open your eyes

Practice Guidelines:

- Perform this exercise daily for at least one week before moving to the next exercise
- Focus on clearly visualizing or sensing each point along the path
- Don't worry about feeling energy yet—this stage is about creating a clear mental map
- Be patient with yourself—some points may be easier to sense than others

Exercise 2: Awakening the Stations

Purpose: To activate the major energy centers (or "stations") along the Microcosmic Orbit path.

Preparation: Same as Exercise 1

Steps:

1. Begin as in Exercise 1, centering with 9 deep breaths
2. Focus your attention on the lower dantian for 9 breaths
3. Move your attention to the perineum (Huiyin point) and focus there for 6 breaths
4. Imagine this point warming and activating, perhaps visualizing it as a small pearl of light
5. Sequentially bring this same focused attention to each major point along the orbit:
   - Sacral center (3 inches below the navel on the spine): 6 breaths
   - Mingmen point (opposite the navel on the spine): 6 breaths
   - Heart center on the back (between shoulder blades): 6 breaths
   - Jade Pillow (at the base of the skull): 6 breaths
   - Crown point (Baihui): 6 breaths
   - Third eye center: 6 breaths
   - Throat center: 6 breaths
   - Heart center (front): 6 breaths
   - Solar plexus: 6 breaths
   - Lower dantian: 9 breaths
6. At each point, use one of these techniques to help activate the center:
   - Visualize a pearl of light growing brighter
   - Imagine a flower opening
   - Simply feel warmth or tingling sensations
7. After completing the circuit, rest in the lower dantian for 3-5 minutes
8. Close by rubbing your palms and smoothing your energy field as in Exercise 1

Practice Guidelines:

- Practice this exercise daily for 1-2 weeks
- Some points may feel more active than others—this is normal
- If you feel uncomfortable sensations at any point (beyond mild tingling or warmth), simply move to the next point
- Keep your attention gentle but focused—straining creates tension that blocks energy

Exercise 3: Circulating the Light

Purpose: To guide qi through the complete Microcosmic Orbit.

Preparation: Same as previous exercises

Steps:

1. Begin with 9 centering breaths
2. Focus on your lower dantian for 12 breaths, until you feel a sense of warmth and gathering energy
3. With an inhalation, draw this energy down to the perineum
4. With the next exhalation, guide the energy up to the sacrum
5. Continue this pattern of using the breath to move energy:
   ○ Inhale: Energy remains stable or gathers at the current point
   ○ Exhale: Energy moves to the next point
6. Move through each point sequentially as in Exercise 2
7. Complete at least 3 full circuits
8. On the final circuit, allow the energy to settle back in the lower dantian
9. Rest in this centered state for 5-10 minutes
10. Close the practice as before

Advanced Variations:

- Once the basic circulation feels comfortable, try guiding the energy with intention alone, without coordinating with the breath
- Experiment with feeling the energy moving as a continuous flow rather than jumping from point to point
- Notice if there are places where the energy seems to stagnate or move slowly—these may indicate blockages to work on

Practice Guidelines:

- Start with 10-15 minutes and gradually extend to 30 minutes
- Practice at least 4-5 times per week
- Be patient—some people feel distinct energy movements quickly, while others develop sensitivity more gradually
- The quality of your attention is more important than the number of circuits completed

Purpose: To identify and release energy blockages along the Microcosmic Orbit.

Preparation: Same as previous exercises

Steps:

1. Complete at least one full circuit as in Exercise 3
2. On the second circuit, move slowly and pay special attention to areas where:
    - The energy seems to move with difficulty
    - You feel discomfort or numbness
    - Your mind tends to wander or lose focus
    - There is tension or emotional response
3. When you identify such an area, pause there and try the following:
    - Focus your attention directly on the blocked area
    - Breathe into the area for 6-9 breaths
    - Visualize the area softening, opening, or becoming more spacious
    - If emotions arise, allow them to be present without judgment
    - Imagine golden light dissolving any stagnation
4. Once the area feels more open, continue the circuit
5. After completing the practice, make note of any persistent blockages for future work
6. Close as in previous exercises

Practice Guidelines:

- Approach blockages with patience and compassion—they often represent stored tension or emotions
- Sometimes blockages take multiple sessions to fully release
- If an area feels particularly charged emotionally, consider complementary practices like journaling or body work
- Honor your process—energetic opening unfolds at its own pace

Part II: Spinal Opening and Breath

Understanding Spinal Energy

In many energy cultivation traditions, the spine is considered the central axis of the human energy system. The Taoists view the spine not just as a physical structure but as the home of the Governing Vessel (Du Mai) and the pathway for the ascending yang energy.

A flexible, open spine allows for:

- Free flow of cerebrospinal fluid
- Healthy nervous system function
- Uninhibited energy circulation
- Proper communication between the brain and all body systems
- Spiritual awakening and higher consciousness

Modern life, with its abundance of sitting and screen time, often leads to spinal compression, tension, and energetic stagnation. The following exercises help restore the spine's natural alignment and energy flow through conscious breath and movement.

Exercises for Spinal Opening

Exercise 5: Spinal Breathing Awareness

Purpose: To develop awareness of the relationship between breath and spinal energy.

Preparation:

- Find a comfortable seated position with your spine naturally straight
- You may sit on a chair, meditation cushion, or against a wall for support
- Wear loose, comfortable clothing

Steps:

1. Place your hands on your knees, palms down
2. Close your eyes and take 5 natural breaths
3. Bring your attention to the base of your spine at the tailbone
4. As you inhale, imagine your breath entering through the base of your spine
5. Feel this breath-energy rising up through your spine to the crown of your head
6. As you exhale, feel the energy descending back down your spine to the tailbone
7. Continue this visualization for 9 breath cycles
8. On the next round, add these refinements:

- o As you inhale and energy rises, imagine your spine gently lengthening
- o As you exhale and energy descends, allow your spine to remain long (avoid collapsing)
9. Continue for another 9 breath cycles
10. In the final round, add awareness of the spaces between the vertebrae:
   - o As you inhale, imagine these spaces expanding slightly
   - o As you exhale, maintain this spaciousness
11. Complete 9 more breath cycles
12. Rest in natural breathing for 2 minutes
13. Slowly open your eyes

Practice Guidelines:

- Focus on smooth, even breath—avoid forcing or straining
- The visualization should be gentle and light, not rigid
- If your mind wanders, simply return to the breath and spinal awareness
- Practice daily for 5-10 minutes

Exercise 6: Spinal Wave

Purpose: To release tension and blockages along the spine through gentle, conscious movement.

Preparation:

- Find a comfortable seated position on the edge of a chair or cushion
- Ensure your feet are flat on the floor if using a chair
- Allow your spine to be free of support

Steps:

1. Place your hands on your thighs or knees
2. Take 5 deep breaths, relaxing your shoulders and jaw
3. Slightly tuck your chin and round your upper back, creating a C-curve
4. Slowly begin to roll backward, vertebra by vertebra, starting from the base of your skull
5. Continue rolling back until your spine is slightly arched (avoid extreme extension)
6. Then begin the forward wave:
   - o Tuck your tailbone slightly
   - o Roll forward vertebra by vertebra, from the base of your spine upward

      o Allow your head to hang forward at the end of the movement
7. Continue these slow, deliberate waves up and down the spine
8. Coordinate with your breath:
      o Inhale as you arch backward
      o Exhale as you round forward
9. Complete 9-12 full cycles
10. Return to a neutral spine position
11. Sit quietly and notice the sensations along your spine
12. Gently twist to each side to release any remaining tension

Refinements:

- Move as slowly as possible to increase awareness
- Imagine your breath massaging each vertebra as you move
- Notice any areas of stiffness or resistance, and bring particular attention to these areas without forcing
- Allow sounds or sighs to emerge naturally as tension releases

Practice Guidelines:

- Practice daily, ideally in the morning or after long periods of sitting
- Start with 3-5 minutes and gradually increase to 10 minutes
- This exercise can be done multiple times throughout the day as needed
- If you have spinal injuries or conditions, consult a healthcare provider first and modify as needed

Exercise 7: Spinal Cord Breathing

Purpose: To awaken and purify the central channel of energy along the spine.

Preparation:

- Find a comfortable seated meditation posture
- Ensure your spine is naturally aligned
- You may sit against a wall if needed for support

Steps:

1. Close your eyes and take 9 deep, relaxing breaths
2. Bring your attention to the base of your spine
3. Visualize your spinal cord as a hollow tube of light

4. For the first round of 9 breaths:
   - Inhale and imagine cool, purifying energy entering through the base of your spine
   - Feel this energy rising through the spinal cord to the crown of your head
   - Exhale and visualize the energy continuing over the crown and down the front of your body
   - Complete the Microcosmic Orbit circuit back to the base of the spine
5. For the second round of 9 breaths:
   - Inhale and visualize the energy entering through the crown of your head
   - Feel it descending through the spinal cord to the base of your spine
   - Exhale and continue the circuit up the front of your body
   - Complete the orbit back to the crown
6. For the third round of 9 breaths:
   - Inhale and imagine energy entering simultaneously from both the crown and the base of the spine
   - Feel these two streams meeting at the heart level
   - Exhale and visualize the energy expanding outward from your heart in all directions
   - On the next inhale, gather the energy back to the spine and continue
7. After completing all three rounds, rest with your awareness at your lower dantian
8. Sit quietly for 3-5 minutes, observing any sensations throughout your body

Refinements:

- Visualize the energy as clear light, golden nectar, or whatever imagery resonates with you
- If you encounter resistance or blockages, breathe into them with patience
- Notice the quality of energy in different sections of your spine
- Allow your breath to become progressively more subtle as you continue

Practice Guidelines:

- Practice 3-4 times per week, preferably not immediately before bed as it can be energizing
- Begin with 10-15 minutes and extend to 20-30 minutes as comfortable
- This practice can generate significant energy—if you feel overwhelmed, ground yourself by focusing on your lower dantian or the soles of your feet

- Journal about your experiences after practice

Understanding Energy Cultivation Through the Hands

The hands contain major energy points connected to the heart, pericardium, and triple heater meridians. They are natural transmitters and receivers of qi. Learning to sense and manipulate energy between your hands develops several important skills:

- Increased sensitivity to subtle energy
- The ability to direct qi with intention
- A tangible experience of energy as a real phenomenon
- The capacity to condense and expand energy
- Skills that transfer to healing applications

This practice is often the first time many students have a concrete, undeniable experience of qi as something more than theoretical. The following exercises progressively develop your ability to sense, gather, and direct energy using your hands.

Exercises for Energy Ball Cultivation

Exercise 8: Awakening Hand Sensitivity

Purpose: To increase awareness of energy sensations in the palms and fingers.

Preparation:

- Find a comfortable seated position
- Ensure you won't be disturbed for 15-20 minutes
- Remove watches, bracelets, or rings if possible

Steps:

1. Rub your palms together vigorously for 15-20 seconds until they feel warm
2. Hold your palms facing each other, about 8-10 inches apart
3. Close your eyes and take 3 deep breaths
4. Slowly begin to move your hands closer together, stopping about 4-6 inches apart
5. With focused awareness, notice any sensations in your palms and fingers:

- o Tingling
- o Warmth
- o Pulsing
- o Magnetism (either attracting or repelling)
- o Pressure or density
- o Coolness

6. After 1-2 minutes, slowly move your hands farther apart (10-12 inches)
7. Again, pay close attention to the sensations
8. Move your hands closer and farther apart 3 more times, noting how the sensations change with distance
9. Rest with your hands about 6 inches apart for 3 minutes, maintaining gentle attention on the sensations
10. To finish, rub your palms together again and then rest them on your knees

Refinements:

- Keep your attention gentle but focused—trying too hard can block sensitivity
- Accept whatever sensations arise without judgment—different people experience energy in different ways
- If you have trouble sensing anything, try smaller movements or closing your eyes to enhance focus
- Experiment with slightly different hand positions—fingers spread vs. together, palms directly facing vs. slightly angled

Practice Guidelines:

- Practice daily for 5-10 minutes
- Morning or evening practice often yields the best results
- Avoid practicing right after heavy meals or when extremely tired
- Be patient—sensitivity develops gradually for most people

Exercise 9: Forming the Energy Ball

Purpose: To gather and condense qi into a palpable energy formation between the hands.

Preparation: Same as Exercise 8

Steps:

1. Begin by rubbing your palms together vigorously
2. Hold your hands about 10 inches apart, palms facing each other
3. Close your eyes and take 5 deep, relaxing breaths
4. Imagine you are holding a small ball of light or energy between your palms
5. As you inhale, visualize energy flowing into this ball from the universe around you
6. As you exhale, imagine energy flowing from your heart center out through your arms and into the ball
7. Continue this visualization for 9 breath cycles
8. Now, begin to slowly move your hands closer together (to about 4-6 inches apart)
9. Feel the energy ball becoming more condensed and concentrated
10. Hold this position for 9 more breaths, continuing to feed energy into the ball
11. Gradually begin to shape the energy by:
    o Slightly rotating your hands
    o Gently pressing inward as if compressing the ball
    o Moving your hands in small circles while maintaining awareness of the center
12. Notice how the sensations between your palms intensify or change
13. After 3-5 minutes of working with the ball, hold your hands still again
14. For the final 9 breaths:
    o Inhale and feel the ball stabilizing
    o Exhale and sense its distinct boundaries
15. To conclude, you can either:
    o Slowly expand the ball until it dissipates into your energy field
    o Bring the ball to your lower dantian and imagine absorbing it there
    o Place your palms on your knees with the energy absorbed into your palms

Refinements:

- Experiment with different sizes of energy balls, from as small as a marble to as large as a basketball
- Try varying the density—sometimes create a very condensed, compact ball, other times a lighter, more expansive one
- Notice if the energy has temperature, color, or texture in your awareness
- With practice, try to maintain awareness of the ball even with your eyes open

Practice Guidelines:

- Practice for 10-15 minutes daily
- As your sensitivity increases, reduce the initial hand rubbing—eventually you'll be able to form the ball directly
- Be aware that your energy levels may affect your perception—notice how the experience differs when you're tired versus energized
- Consider practicing outdoors in natural settings to experience how different environments affect the energy

Exercise 10: Dynamic Energy Ball Work

Purpose: To develop the ability to manipulate, transform, and direct qi through the energy ball.

Preparation: Same as previous exercises

Steps:

1. Create an energy ball between your hands as in Exercise 9
2. Once you have a clear sensation of the ball, begin these dynamic practices:
3. Expansion and Contraction (3 minutes):
   - Inhale and slowly move your hands farther apart, feeling the ball expand while maintaining its integrity
   - Exhale and bring your hands closer, condensing the energy
   - Repeat 9 times, noting how far you can expand before losing sensation of the ball
4. Energy Ball Bounce (2 minutes):
   - Gently "bounce" the ball by making small up and down movements with your hands
   - Feel the resilience and elasticity of the energy
   - Experiment with different rhythms and intensities
5. Temperature Transformation (3 minutes):
   - Visualize the ball becoming intensely warm for 9 breaths
   - Then transform it to cool energy for 9 breaths
   - Notice which temperature feels more natural or powerful for you
6. Energy Transfer (4 minutes):
   - Hold the ball primarily between your right hand (below) and left hand (above)
   - Gradually shift the ball to between your left hand (below) and right hand (above)

- Continue transferring the ball from side to side, maintaining its integrity
- Feel how the energy moves through your body during the transfer

7. Integration (3 minutes):
    - Bring the ball to your lower dantian (about 1.5 inches below your navel)
    - Place both hands over this area
    - Visualize the ball of energy merging with your dantian
    - Feel this energy spreading throughout your body

8. Completion:
    - Place your hands on your knees, palms down
    - Take 9 deep breaths, feeling yourself fully integrated and centered
    - Gently open your eyes

Advanced Variations:

- Try forming the energy ball with only one hand
- Practice maintaining awareness of the energy ball while walking slowly
- Experiment with projecting energy from the ball toward objects (plants often respond well)
- Form the ball and then use it to scan your body for areas of imbalance

Practice Guidelines:

- Practice the complete sequence 2-3 times weekly
- Additionally, incorporate individual elements into daily practice
- As your sensitivity develops, reduce the time spent on basic elements and expand time on advanced variations
- Keep a journal of your experiences, noting patterns in energy quality

Integration and Further Practice

The three practices in this chapter—Microcosmic Orbit, Spinal Opening, and Energy Ball Work—complement each other beautifully. The Energy Ball practice develops your ability to sense and direct qi, making your Microcosmic Orbit practice more tangible. The Spinal Opening exercises clear blockages in the Governing Vessel, enhancing flow in the orbit.

For optimal development, consider this weekly practice schedule:

- Daily: 10-minute Spinal Opening (morning)

- 3-4 times weekly: 20-minute Microcosmic Orbit
- 2-3 times weekly: 15-minute Energy Ball practice
- Once weekly: An extended session combining all three practices (45-60 minutes)

As these practices become more familiar, you'll naturally discover how to adapt and integrate them according to your unique energy system and needs. Listen to your body's wisdom and allow your practice to evolve organically.

Remember that energy work is cumulative—consistent practice over time yields much greater results than occasional intensive sessions. Even 10-15 minutes daily will produce significant changes in your energy awareness and flow over the course of months.

Common Experiences and Troubleshooting

As you work with these practices, you may encounter various sensations and experiences. Here are some common ones and how to approach them:

Tingling, Warmth, or Magnetic Sensations: These are normal and positive signs of energy movement. Simply observe them without attachment.

Spontaneous Body Movements: Small trembling, swaying, or involuntary movements often indicate energy releasing blockages. Allow these unless they become disruptive.

Emotional Releases: Tears, laughter, or sudden emotions may arise as energy moves through blocked areas. Allow these expressions without judgment.

Difficulty Sensing Energy: This is common, especially initially. Focus on the physical sensations of breath and posture, and energy awareness will develop gradually.

Falling Asleep: If you consistently feel sleepy during practice, try practicing at a different time of day, sitting in a more upright posture, or taking a short walk beforehand.

Discomfort or Pain: Mild discomfort as energy moves through tight areas is normal, but actual pain indicates you should adjust your practice. Reduce intensity, change position, or focus elsewhere.

Energy Overwhelm: If you feel anxious, jittery, or overstimulated, ground your energy by focusing on your feet or lower dantian, reduce practice time, and consider adding more physical exercise to your routine.

Remember that each person's energy system is unique. Trust your experience and adapt these practices to serve your individual path of development.

The practices in this chapter form the foundation of energy cultivation in the internal arts. Through diligent practice, you'll develop:

1. Clear energy pathways through the Microcosmic Orbit
2. An open, responsive spine that serves as a conduit for higher energies
3. The ability to sense, gather, and direct qi for healing and spiritual development

As your practice deepens, you'll discover that these techniques not only transform your energy body but also bring profound changes to your physical health, emotional balance, and spiritual awareness. The subtle becomes tangible, and what once seemed esoteric becomes your lived experience.

In the next chapter, we'll explore how to extend these foundational practices to work with the energy of the five elements and their corresponding organ systems, further refining your internal energy circulation and balance.

Reflection Questions

Before moving to the next chapter, consider these questions:

1. What sensations do you most consistently feel during energy practice? How have they evolved since you began?
2. Which areas of your body seem most responsive to energy work? Which areas seem most blocked or difficult to sense?
3. How has your breathing changed since beginning these practices?
4. What effects have you noticed in your daily life since working with these energy cultivation techniques?
5. Which of the three main practices resonates most strongly with you, and why?

Take time to journal about your experiences and insights, creating a record of your unique journey with these ancient and powerful practices.

"The wise student practices diligently yet remains patient, knowing that just as water gradually shapes stone, consistent energy work inevitably transforms the being."

Workbook: Channel Opening and Flow

Journal Reflection

Contemplate: How has your relationship with your body's energy flow changed through these practices? What insights or shifts have emerged as you work with your channels and breath?

Your Reflection:

_____

Practice Tracker

Track your Microcosmic Orbit, Spinal Opening, and Energy Ball practices throughout the week.

Date	Practice Type	Duration (min)	Felt Sensations	Areas of Blockage or Flow

Microcosmic Orbit Practice Log

Describe your experience during Microcosmic Orbit sessions. Include sensations, flow quality, and any challenges or breakthroughs.

Spinal Opening & Breathwork Log

Note physical and energetic shifts during spinal practices. What changed in your posture, awareness, or breath?

Energy Ball Practice Log

What did you feel between your hands? How did the energy respond to your intention? Note size, texture, and effects of the energy ball.

Reflection Questions

1. What sensations do you most consistently feel during energy practice? How have they evolved?

_____

2. Which areas of your body seem most responsive to energy work? Which areas feel blocked?

_____

3. How has your breathing changed since beginning these practices?

_____

4. What changes have you noticed in your emotional or mental state?

_____

5. Which of the three main practices resonates most deeply with you, and why?

_____

Chapter 6: Jing to Qi – Sexual Energy and Vitality

In the vast landscape of traditional Chinese medicine and Taoist cultivation practices, the understanding and refinement of our vital energies stands as a cornerstone of health, longevity, and spiritual development. This chapter explores the profound connection between our primordial essence (Jing), vital energy (Qi), and the practices that allow us to transform and conserve these precious resources.

The ancient Taoists discovered that our sexual energy—far from being merely for procreation or pleasure—represents one of our most potent resources for healing, creativity, and spiritual transformation. When properly understood and cultivated, this energy becomes the foundation for robust health, mental clarity, emotional balance, and extended vitality throughout our lives.

In this chapter, we will explore the practical wisdom of Jing conservation, the arts of Yang Sheng (nourishing life), and the foundational concepts of inner alchemy that have been refined over thousands of years. These teachings bridge the gap between sexuality and spirituality, offering a holistic approach to enhancing your vital force that extends far beyond the physical realm.

The Three Treasures: Jing, Qi, and Shen

Before delving into specific practices, it's essential to understand the framework of the Three Treasures, which form the energetic foundation of Taoist internal arts:

1. **Jing (Essence)**: The densest form of energy in the body, often associated with sexual fluids and reproductive essence, but more broadly representing our constitutional strength and genetic inheritance. Jing is like the wax of a candle—finite unless replenished and conserved.
2. **Qi (Vital Energy)**: The dynamic life force that animates the body and circulates through the meridian system. Qi is like the flame of the candle—visible, active, warming, and constantly in motion.
3. **Shen (Spirit)**: The most refined energy, associated with consciousness, mental clarity, and spiritual awareness. Shen is like the light emanating from the candle—radiant, illuminating, and far-reaching.

The art of internal cultivation involves transforming denser energies into more refined ones—specifically, learning to transform Jing into Qi, and eventually Qi into Shen. This alchemical process is at the heart of Taoist longevity practices.

Jing Conservation and Transformation

Understanding Jing Essence

Jing is our most fundamental energy reserve. In Taoist terms, we receive pre-natal Jing from our parents at conception, while post-natal Jing is generated throughout our lives from food, air, water, and healthy lifestyle practices. Traditional wisdom holds that excessive loss of Jing—particularly through sexual activity without proper understanding of energy management—can deplete our vital reserves and accelerate aging.

However, this doesn't mean sexual abstinence is the answer. Rather, it points to the importance of learning how to engage with our sexual energy wisely, using specific practices to circulate, refine, and conserve this powerful force.

Exercise 1: Jing Awareness Practice

Purpose: To develop sensitivity to your Jing levels and understand how different activities affect your essential energy.

Duration: 10-15 minutes daily for one week

Steps:

1. Sit comfortably with your spine erect and eyes closed.
2. Place your hands on your lower abdomen, just below your navel.
3. Breathe deeply and slowly, drawing your awareness to this area (known as the lower Dantian).
4. Observe the sensations of warmth, fullness, or emptiness in this region.
5. Reflect on your energy levels over the past 24 hours, noting activities that either depleted or enhanced your sense of core vitality.
6. After 5-10 minutes of this awareness practice, gently massage your lower abdomen in a clockwise direction for 36 rotations.
7. Complete the practice with three deep breaths, drawing energy into your lower Dantian.

Integration: Keep a daily journal noting your observations about activities, foods, emotions, or interactions that either strengthen or deplete your Jing. Look for patterns over the week.

Exercise 2: The Inner Smile to the Kidneys

Purpose: The kidneys are considered the storehouse of Jing in traditional Chinese medicine. This practice helps to nourish and replenish kidney energy.

Duration: 10-15 minutes

Steps:

1. Sit comfortably and relax your body with several deep breaths.
2. Generate a genuine feeling of smiling, recalling a pleasant memory if needed.
3. Allow this smile to radiate from your face down to your kidneys (located at the back of your body at waist level).
4. Visualize your kidneys as two dark blue pools of water, becoming refreshed and revitalized by your smiling energy.
5. Imagine a cool, blue light filling your kidneys, restoring and replenishing them.
6. As you inhale, feel the kidney energy being purified; as you exhale, feel any staleness or fatigue being released.
7. Continue for 5-10 minutes, then collect the energy at your lower Dantian.

Integration: Practice this whenever you feel depleted, especially after stressful interactions or excessive mental work.

Exercise 3: Sexual Energy Circulation – The Microcosmic Orbit Basics

Purpose: To learn to circulate sexual energy rather than expending it, transforming Jing into Qi.

Duration: 15-20 minutes

Steps:

1. Sit comfortably with your spine straight.
2. Focus your attention on your perineum (the area between your genitals and anus).

3. As you inhale, draw energy from this sexual center up your spine.
4. Visualize this energy as a warm, golden light traveling up through your tailbone, along your spine, and to the top of your head.
5. As you exhale, guide this energy down the front of your body—through your face, throat, chest, and abdomen—returning to the perineum.
6. Continue this circulation for 9-36 complete breaths.
7. To conclude, collect the energy at your lower Dantian by placing your hands there and circling 36 times.

Important Note: If you feel any uncomfortable sensations such as headache, dizziness, or excessive heat, stop immediately and focus on your lower Dantian or soles of your feet to ground the energy.

Integration: This practice can be especially beneficial before or after situations where sexual energy is activated, helping to transform it into available Qi for your body's use rather than expending it.

The Lifestyle of Yang Sheng (Nourishing Life)

Yang Sheng translates as "nourishing life" and encompasses the comprehensive Taoist approach to cultivating health and longevity through daily practices and lifestyle choices. This ancient wisdom provides practical guidance for maintaining and enhancing our vital energies.

The Five Pillars of Yang Sheng

1. **Nutrition**: Eating for Jing and Qi enhancement
2. **Rest and Activity**: Balancing exertion with recovery
3. **Emotional Harmony**: Managing stress and cultivating positive emotions
4. **Environmental Awareness**: Creating supportive surroundings
5. **Sexual Wisdom**: Practices for energetic cultivation

Exercise 4: Jing-Nourishing Nutrition Awareness

Purpose: To identify and incorporate foods that support Jing replenishment.

Duration: 3-day food awareness practice

Steps:

1. For three days, incorporate at least one Jing-nourishing food from each category below:
   o **Black Foods**: Black beans, black sesame seeds, black rice, blackberries
   o **Kidney-Supporting Foods**: Walnuts, chestnuts, bone broth, sardines
   o **Mineral-Rich Foods**: Seaweeds, dark leafy greens, spirulina, nettle tea
   o **Clean Water**: Hydrate adequately with filtered water
2. Before consuming these foods, take a moment to set an intention for nourishing your deep vital essence.
3. Eat mindfully, chewing thoroughly and appreciating the nourishment these foods provide.
4. Note how different foods affect your energy levels, particularly your sense of deep, constitutional strength.

Integration: Based on your observations, create a sustainable nutrition plan that regularly incorporates Jing-supportive foods.

Exercise 5: Restoration Practice – The Inner Sanctuary

Purpose: To create dedicated time for deep rest that allows Jing to regenerate.

Duration: 20-30 minutes

Steps:

1. Create a quiet, comfortable space where you won't be disturbed.
2. Lie down on your back with your knees slightly bent or supported by a pillow.
3. Place one hand on your lower abdomen and one on your heart center.
4. Close your eyes and take several deep, slow breaths.
5. With each exhale, allow your body to sink more deeply into relaxation.
6. Visualize yourself in a peaceful natural setting—perhaps a secluded garden, forest grove, or mountainside.
7. In this inner sanctuary, imagine your body being infused with regenerative energy from the earth beneath you.
8. Remain in this state of receptive restoration for 15-25 minutes.
9. Before concluding, mentally scan your body and express gratitude for this time of renewal.

10. Slowly reawaken your body with gentle movements and stretches before getting up.

Integration: Schedule this restoration practice 2-3 times weekly, particularly during periods of stress or intensive activity. Consider it an investment in your vital energy bank account.

Exercise 6: Environmental Energy Audit

Purpose: To identify and enhance the energetic quality of your living spaces.

Duration: 1 hour plus implementation time

Steps:

1. Walk through each room of your home or workspace with a notebook.
2. In each space, pause and notice:
   - How does this space make you feel energetically?
   - Is there adequate fresh air and natural light?
   - What is the noise level and sound quality?
   - Is there clutter that restricts energy flow?
   - Are there elements that nourish your senses (pleasant textures, colors, scents)?
3. Rate each space on a scale of 1-10 for how well it supports your vital energy.
4. For spaces scoring below 7, identify three specific changes you could make to improve the energetic quality:
   - Adding plants or natural elements
   - Improving air circulation or light
   - Reducing clutter or reorganizing
   - Incorporating uplifting colors or artwork
   - Enhancing comfort with better seating or supportive furniture
5. Implement at least one improvement in each space over the next week.

Integration: Schedule a monthly mini-audit to maintain awareness of how your environment affects your energy and make adjustments as needed.

Inner Elixir Formation Basics

The cultivation of inner elixir (Nei Dan) represents the most refined aspect of Taoist energy work. This involves sophisticated practices to purify, refine, and circulate our internal energies. While mastery requires guidance from an experienced teacher, we can begin with foundational practices that prepare the energetic system.

Exercise 7: Lower Dantian Breathing

Purpose: To connect with and strengthen your energy center, preparing the foundation for inner elixir work.

Duration: 10-15 minutes daily

Steps:

1. Sit comfortably with your spine naturally erect.
2. Place your hands one over the other on your lower abdomen, below your navel.
3. Take several normal breaths, then begin to deepen your breath into your abdomen.
4. With each inhale, gently expand your lower abdomen into your hands.
5. With each exhale, allow your abdomen to softly contract.
6. After establishing this breathing pattern, begin to imagine a golden light gathering in your lower Dantian with each breath.
7. With inhales, visualize this light becoming brighter and more condensed.
8. With exhales, visualize this light becoming more stable and radiant.
9. Continue for 5-10 minutes, gradually extending the practice as you build capacity.
10. To conclude, circulate your hands over your lower abdomen 36 times clockwise.

Integration: This practice can be done daily, ideally in the morning to establish your energy for the day and in the evening to restore your core vitality.

Exercise 8: The Internal Elements Balancing

Purpose: To harmonize the five elemental energies within the body, creating the conditions for inner elixir formation.

Duration: 15-20 minutes

Steps:

1. Sit comfortably and establish deep, relaxed breathing.
2. Begin by connecting with the Water element in your kidneys and bladder:
   - Visualize deep blue or black energy here
   - Feel a quality of flowing depth and stillness
   - Inhale cool, purifying energy; exhale any fear or depletion
3. Move to the Wood element in your liver and gallbladder:
   - Visualize vibrant green energy
   - Feel qualities of flexibility, growth, and new beginnings
   - Inhale expanding vitality; exhale stagnation or frustration
4. Continue to the Fire element in your heart and small intestine:
   - Visualize bright red or purple light
   - Feel qualities of joy, warmth, and connection
   - Inhale loving warmth; exhale anxiety or excessive heat
5. Move to the Earth element in your spleen and stomach:
   - Visualize golden yellow energy
   - Feel qualities of centeredness, nourishment, and stability
   - Inhale supportive strength; exhale worry or overthinking
6. Finish with the Metal element in your lungs and large intestine:
   - Visualize white or silver light
   - Feel qualities of clarity, precision, and letting go
   - Inhale pure, crisp energy; exhale grief or attachment
7. To conclude, visualize all five elemental energies flowing in harmony throughout your body, creating a balanced internal environment.

Integration: Practice weekly to maintain elemental balance, or whenever you feel particularly affected by one element's imbalance (e.g., excessive worry, anger, or anxiety).

Exercise 9: The Three Treasures Meditation

Purpose: To experience the relationship between Jing, Qi, and Shen and begin the process of refinement.

Duration: 20-30 minutes

Steps:

1. Find a quiet place and sit in a comfortable meditation posture.
2. Begin with several minutes of deep abdominal breathing to settle your mind and energy.

3. Bring your awareness to your lower Dantian, the storehouse of Jing.
   - Visualize a deep blue essence here, like the depths of the ocean
   - Feel its substantial, dense quality
   - With each breath, sense this essence becoming slightly warmer and more fluid
4. Gradually visualize this essence beginning to transform into Qi:
   - See tendrils of misty energy rising from the dense Jing
   - This mist begins to circulate through your torso and limbs
   - It carries a feeling of activation and movement
5. Guide this Qi up to your middle Dantian at your heart center:
   - Here the energy becomes refined further
   - It transforms from mist to a clear, golden light
   - This light pulses with your heartbeat
6. Finally, guide the refined energy to your upper Dantian:
   - Here the golden light transforms into a brilliant, crystal-clear radiance
   - This is Shen, your spiritual energy
   - Experience its qualities of clarity, spaciousness, and awareness
7. Allow your attention to rest in this clear awareness for 5-10 minutes.
8. To conclude, visualize this refined energy flowing back down through your body, blessing and harmonizing all your systems before settling back into your lower Dantian.

Integration: This meditation provides a conceptual and experiential map of the alchemical transformation at the heart of Taoist practice. With regular practice, you may begin to feel these processes happening naturally.

Sexual Energy Practices for Vitality

While detailed sexual cultivation practices require personalized instruction, we can explore some foundational approaches that help redirect and refine sexual energy for overall vitality.

The Basis of Sexual Energy Transformation

The key principle in Taoist sexual practices is not suppression but transformation. Rather than losing sexual essence through unaware expression, practitioners learn to:

1. **Circulate**: Direct sexual energy through the body's channels
2. **Purify**: Refine the quality of this energy

3. **Store**: Conserve this energy in the appropriate centers
4. **Apply**: Use this refined energy for healing, creativity, and spiritual development

Exercise 10: Ovarian/Testicular Breathing

Purpose: To enhance sexual energy and redirect it for vitality.

Duration: 10-15 minutes

Steps:

For those with female anatomy:

1. Sit comfortably with your spine erect.
2. Place your hands on your lower abdomen, below your navel.
3. Bring your awareness to your ovaries.
4. As you inhale, imagine drawing energy from your ovaries up to your kidneys.
5. As you exhale, allow this energy to flow down to your lower Dantian.
6. Continue this circulation for 9-18 breaths.
7. Then begin to draw the energy up from the lower Dantian, up the spine to the crown of your head, and down the front of your body back to the lower Dantian (the Microcosmic Orbit).
8. Complete 9-18 cycles of this fuller circulation.

For those with male anatomy:

1. Sit comfortably with your spine erect.
2. Place your hands on your lower abdomen, below your navel.
3. Bring your awareness to your testicles.
4. As you inhale, imagine drawing energy from your testicles up to your kidneys.
5. As you exhale, allow this energy to flow down to your lower Dantian.
6. Continue this circulation for 9-18 breaths.
7. Then begin to draw the energy up from the lower Dantian, up the spine to the crown of your head, and down the front of your body back to the lower Dantian (the Microcosmic Orbit).
8. Complete 9-18 cycles of this fuller circulation.

Integration: This practice can be particularly helpful during times of sexual arousal, helping to circulate and refine this energy rather than expending it.

Exercise 11: The Deer Exercise

Purpose: An ancient Taoist practice for strengthening sexual organs and transforming sexual energy.

Duration: 5-10 minutes

Steps:

For those with female anatomy:

1. Stand with feet shoulder-width apart, knees slightly bent.
2. Place your hands on your lower abdomen.
3. Contract your perineum and vaginal muscles, holding for 3-9 seconds.
4. Release the contraction and relax completely.
5. Repeat for 9-36 repetitions, gradually building capacity over time.
6. With each contraction, visualize drawing healing energy into your reproductive organs.
7. With each release, visualize any stagnant energy being cleared away.
8. After completing the repetitions, massage your lower abdomen clockwise 36 times to gather and store the energy.

For those with male anatomy:

1. Stand with feet shoulder-width apart, knees slightly bent.
2. Place your hands on your lower abdomen.
3. Contract your perineum and scrotal muscles while gently drawing your testicles upward, holding for 3-9 seconds.
4. Release the contraction and relax completely.
5. Repeat for 9-36 repetitions, gradually building capacity over time.
6. With each contraction, visualize drawing healing energy into your reproductive organs.
7. With each release, visualize any stagnant energy being cleared away.
8. After completing the repetitions, massage your lower abdomen clockwise 36 times to gather and store the energy.

Integration: Practice once daily, ideally in the morning or evening. This exercise strengthens the physical organs while also helping to refine and direct sexual energy.

The Path of Integration

The journey of transforming Jing to Qi represents one of the most powerful aspects of Taoist internal practice. By understanding the precious nature of our essential energy and learning methods to conserve, transform, and apply it wisely, we establish the foundation for extraordinary vitality and longevity.

Remember that these practices work gradually and cumulatively. Consistency is far more important than intensity. Even five minutes of focused practice daily will yield greater benefits than occasional longer sessions.

As you integrate these practices into your life, approach them with respect, patience, and playful curiosity. Pay attention to how your energy responds and make adjustments accordingly. Each person's energetic system is unique, so honor your own experience and trust the innate wisdom of your body.

The ultimate goal is not just the preservation of physical vitality, but the gradual refinement of your entire being—transforming the physical into the energetic, the energetic into the spiritual, and ultimately discovering the integrated wholeness that has been your birthright all along.

In the next chapter, we will explore how these energetic foundations support higher spiritual awareness and consciousness transformation.

Workbook: Jing to Qi – Sexual Energy and Vitality

This workbook is designed to help you integrate the concepts and practices from the chapter into your daily life. Through consistent practice, self-reflection, and tracking, you'll develop a deeper understanding of your own energy systems and how to cultivate greater vitality.

Use this workbook as your companion on this journey of energy cultivation. Be honest with yourself in your reflections, patient with your progress, and compassionate toward your challenges. Remember that this work is deeply personal—there is no standard timeline or "correct" experience. Your body and energy system are unique, and your practice should honor that individuality.

Section 1: Practice Log – Dantian Breathing & Microcosmic Orbit

Weekly Practice Schedule

Use this schedule to plan and track your daily practices. Aim for consistency rather than duration—even 5-10 minutes daily will yield cumulative benefits.

Day	Practice Duration Time of Day Notes
Monday	
Tuesday	
Wednesday	
Thursday	
Friday	
Saturday	
Sunday	

Lower Dantian Breathing Log

Track your experience with the Lower Dantian Breathing practice:

Date: _____

Duration: _____

Physical sensations observed:

Quality of breath (shallow/deep, smooth/jerky, etc.):

Sensations in the lower Dantian area:

Challenges encountered:

Insights or breakthroughs:

Microcosmic Orbit Practice Log

Track your experience with the Microcosmic Orbit circulation:

Date: _____

Duration: _____

Number of complete circuits: _____

Areas where energy flowed easily:

Areas where energy seemed blocked or stagnant:

Sensations along the governing vessel (back channel):

Sensations along the conception vessel (front channel):

Overall energy state after practice:

Monthly Practice Review

At the end of each month, take time to review your practice:

Month: _____

Total number of practice sessions: _____

Average duration per session: _____

Most consistent practice (which exercise did you do most regularly?):

Most noticeable changes in energy awareness:

Challenges to consistent practice:

Strategies to overcome these challenges next month:

Goals for next month's practice:

Section 2: Reflective Journal – "How Do I Experience Energy Now?"

Use these journaling prompts to deepen your awareness of energy in your body and life. Try to write in this section at least once per week.

Energy Mapping Exercise

Draw a simple outline of your body and use colors, symbols, or words to indicate:

- Areas of strong energy/vitality
- Areas of depletion or stagnation
- Areas of tension or blockage
- Areas of warmth or coolness
- Areas of natural flow or movement

After completing your map, write a brief description of your current energy state:

Date: _____

Overall energy level today (1-10): _____

Describe the quality of your energy today (e.g., scattered, focused, heavy, light, etc.):

Activities/situations that enhanced my energy this week:

Activities/situations that depleted my energy this week:

Changes I've noticed in my energy since beginning these practices:

Questions arising about my energy cultivation:

Current relationship with sexual energy (circle or note what applies):

- Depleting
- Neutral
- Nourishing
- Confusing
- Transformative
- Other: _____

Ways I've noticed sexual energy affecting my overall vitality:

Practices that have helped me work with sexual energy constructively:

Challenges in working with sexual energy:

Insights about the connection between sexual energy and creativity/vitality:

Three Treasures Reflection

Take some time to reflect on your experience of each treasure:

Jing (Essence):

- How would I describe my constitutional strength?

- When do I feel most depleted at this deep level?
- What practices help me feel restored at this level?

Qi (Vital Energy):

- How would I describe my day-to-day energy patterns?
- What affects the quality and quantity of my Qi?
- How do I experience Qi movement in my body?

Shen (Spirit):

- How would I describe my mental clarity and spiritual awareness?
- When do I feel most connected to this aspect of myself?
- What practices enhance this dimension of my being?

Section 3: Dietary and Lifestyle Tracker

Jing-Nourishing Foods Tracker

Track your consumption of Jing-supportive foods:

Date	Black Foods	Kidney-Supporting Foods	Mineral-Rich Foods	Water Intake	Notes on Energy Effects

Rate each aspect of your lifestyle on a scale of 1-10 (1 = needs significant improvement, 10 = excellent):

Weekly Assessment Date: _____

Yang Sheng Aspect	Rating (1-10)	Observations	One Improvement to Implement
Nutrition			
Rest & Sleep			
Exercise & Movement			
Emotional Balance			
Environmental Quality			
Sexual Energy Management			
Stress Management			
Social Connections			
Spiritual Practice			

Sleep Quality Tracker

Since sleep is crucial for Jing restoration, track your sleep patterns:

Date	Hours Slept	Sleep Quality (1-10)	Dreams?	Pre-Sleep Routine	Morning Energy

Energy Leakage Assessment

Identify areas where you may be unnecessarily losing vital energy:

Areas to Assess:

Digital/Media Consumption:

- Hours spent daily: _____
- Effect on energy (depleting, neutral, energizing): _____
- One adjustment to make: _____

Emotional Patterns:

- Recurring emotional drains: _____
- Emotional nourishment practices: _____
- One adjustment to make: _____

Social Interactions:

- Energy-depleting relationships: _____
- Energy-enhancing relationships: _____
- One adjustment to make: _____

Physical Environment:

- Areas of disorder/chaos: _____
- Harmonious spaces: _____
- One adjustment to make: _____

Sexual Energy Management:

- Current patterns: _____
- Effect on overall energy: _____
- One adjustment to make: _____

Section 4: Self-Assessment

Use these assessments periodically (perhaps monthly) to track your progress in developing energy awareness and cultivation.

Energy Body Assessment

Rate your awareness and capacity in each area (1 = minimal, 10 = highly developed):

Energy Aspect	Initial Rating	1 Month	3 Months	6 Months
Lower Dantian awareness				
Middle Dantian awareness				
Upper Dantian awareness				
Back channel flow				
Front channel flow				
Ability to direct Qi				
Sexual energy awareness				
Jing conservation skill				
Overall energy management				

Practice Competency Self-Assessment

Rate your competency with each practice (1 = beginner, 10 = proficient):

Practice	Initial Rating	1 Month	3 Months	6 Months
Lower Dantian Breathing				
Microcosmic Orbit				
Inner Smile to Kidneys				
Ovarian/Testicular Breathing				
Deer Exercise				
Three Treasures Meditation				
Elements Balancing				

Use this space to record significant experiences, breakthroughs, or realizations:

Date: _____

Experience/Insight:

Context (during which practice, life situation, etc.):

Effect on understanding or practice:

Section 5: Integration Planning

Daily Integration Plan

Design a sustainable daily routine that incorporates energy practices:

Morning routine:

Midday energy reset:

Evening practice:

Dietary intentions:

Movement/exercise plan:

Weekly Integration Plan

Longer practices (which days, duration):

Rest and restoration focus:

Social energy management:

Environmental energy work:

As seasons change, note adjustments to your practice to align with natural cycles:

Season: _____

Energy qualities of this season: _____

PART III: Shen Gong – Refining Qi into Shen

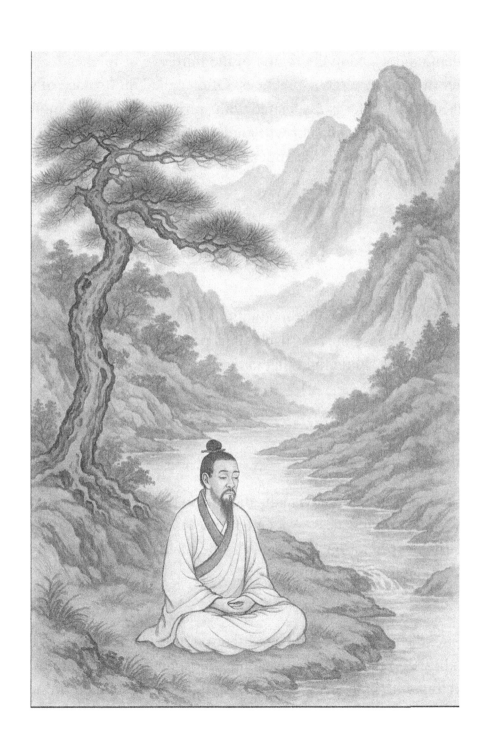

The upper dantian, located in the region of the third eye or forehead, is a vital energy center in Taoist energetic practices. Often called the "palace of spirit" or "crystal palace," this center is associated with spiritual awakening, intuition, and higher consciousness. This chapter will guide you through three powerful practices for awakening and developing the upper dantian: Inner Light meditation, Shen breathing, and third eye activation.

Inner Light Meditation

In Taoist tradition, the Inner Light meditation connects practitioners with the luminous quality of consciousness itself. This practice involves turning awareness inward to perceive the subtle light that naturally emanates within.

Understanding Inner Light

The Inner Light is not merely a visualization but a perception of the subtle radiance that exists within consciousness. Ancient Taoist texts describe this light as the "original spirit" or "primordial awareness" - the fundamental luminosity of being that precedes thought and sensation.

When we quiet the mind and refine our attention, this inner brightness becomes perceptible. Initially, it may appear as gentle phosphenes (light patterns behind closed eyes), but with practice, it can develop into a clear, radiant presence.

The Practice of Inner Light Meditation

Exercise 1: Connecting with Inner Light

Step-by-Step Instructions:

1. Find a quiet space and sit in a comfortable position with your spine straight.

2. Close your eyes and take several deep breaths to settle your mind and body.

3. Bring your attention to the space between your eyebrows (the third eye region).

4. Without straining, gently focus your awareness on this area as if gazing inward.

5. Notice any subtle sensations, warmth, or tingling that may arise.

6. Observe any natural luminosity, colors, or light patterns that may appear behind your closed eyes.

7. Rather than actively visualizing light, adopt a receptive awareness—simply noticing what naturally appears.

8. If your mind wanders, gently return your attention to the third eye region.

9. Continue for 10-15 minutes, gradually extending the duration as you become more familiar with the practice.

10. To conclude, gently bring your awareness back to your whole body, take a few deep breaths, and slowly open your eyes.

Exercise 2: Cultivating the Pearl of Light

Step-by-Step Instructions:

1. Begin as in Exercise 1, establishing a relaxed awareness at the third eye center.

2. As you perceive any natural luminosity, imagine it gradually condensing into a small pearl of light at the center of your forehead.

3. Allow this pearl to grow brighter and more defined with each breath.

4. Inhale and feel the pearl absorbing universal light energy.

5. Exhale and feel the pearl stabilizing and growing more radiant.

6. Maintain a gentle focus on this pearl for 5-10 minutes.

7. Gradually expand the pearl to fill your entire head with luminous awareness.

8. Rest in this expanded light state for another 5-10 minutes.

9. To conclude, visualize the light gradually returning to a pearl size, then dissolving into your third eye center.

10. Take several deep breaths and slowly open your eyes.

Shen Breathing

Shen refers to spirit or consciousness in Taoist tradition. Shen breathing involves using the breath to cultivate and refine spiritual energy in the upper dantian. This practice creates a harmonious relationship between breath, awareness, and spiritual essence.

Understanding Shen Breathing

Unlike regular breathing practices that focus on the physical aspects of breath, Shen breathing emphasizes the relationship between breath and consciousness. The breath becomes a vehicle for spirit, carrying awareness throughout the subtle energy body and particularly to the upper dantian.

By synchronizing breath with attention, we can direct spiritual energy (Shen) to the upper center, refining and awakening its potential.

The Practice of Shen Breathing

Exercise 1: Foundation Shen Breathing

Step-by-Step Instructions:

1. Sit in a comfortable position with your spine straight and shoulders relaxed.

2. Place the tip of your tongue lightly against the roof of your mouth, just behind your front teeth.

3. Close your eyes and bring your awareness to your breath, allowing it to become smooth and even.

4. As you inhale, visualize pure, clear light being drawn up through your spine to your upper dantian.

5. As you exhale, feel this light illuminating and expanding within your forehead area.

6. With each inhalation, silently repeat the word "Shen" or simply think "spirit ascending."

7. With each exhalation, feel your consciousness expanding and brightening.

8. Continue for 10-15 minutes, maintaining a gentle but focused awareness.

9. To conclude, release any visualization and simply rest in awareness for a few minutes.

10. Take three deep breaths and open your eyes.

Exercise 2: Advanced Shen Breathing Circulation

Step-by-Step Instructions:

1. Begin with 5 minutes of foundation Shen breathing to establish the connection.

2. On inhalation, visualize luminous energy rising from your lower dantian (below navel) through your middle dantian (heart) to your upper dantian (forehead).

3. Hold the breath gently for a moment, feeling the three dantians connected by a stream of light.

4. As you exhale, visualize this light radiating outward from your upper dantian in all directions.

5. Continue this breathing pattern, creating a continuous flow of energy from lower to upper centers.

6. After 10-15 cycles, begin to visualize a circular flow: on inhalation, energy rises from lower to upper dantian; on exhalation, it flows down the front of your body back to the lower dantian.

7. Continue this circular breathing for 10-15 minutes.

8. Gradually slow the circulation and allow your breath to return to normal.

9. Rest in simple awareness for a few minutes.

10. Gently massage your face and scalp before opening your eyes.

Activating Third Eye Awareness

The third eye, corresponding to the sixth chakra in yogic traditions and the upper dantian in Taoism, is often described as the seat of intuition, insight, and expanded perception. Activating this center involves refined attention and energetic cultivation.

Understanding Third Eye Awareness

The third eye is not merely a metaphorical concept but a subtle energy center that can be experienced directly. When activated, it enhances intuitive perception, spiritual insight, and may even allow access to non-ordinary states of awareness.

This center bridges the conscious and subconscious minds, facilitating deeper understanding of both inner and outer realities. Regular practice helps purify and awaken this center, leading to greater clarity and spiritual awareness.

The Practice of Third Eye Activation

Exercise 1: Third Eye Sensing

Step-by-Step Instructions:

1. Sit comfortably with your spine straight and eyes closed.

2. Take several deep breaths, relaxing your face, jaw, and forehead.

3. Bring your attention to the space between your eyebrows.

4. Gently press this area with your index finger for a few seconds, then release.

5. Notice any sensations, warmth, or subtle pressure that remains.

6. Without straining, direct your attention to this point as if looking through it rather than at it.

7. Imagine a small window or aperture opening in this area, connecting you to expanded awareness.

8. Breathe naturally, allowing each breath to gently stimulate and awaken this center.

9. If you notice tension, consciously relax your forehead and eyes while maintaining awareness at the third eye center.

10. Practice for 10-15 minutes, gradually building the duration as you become more comfortable.

Exercise 2: Third Eye Energy Cultivation

Step-by-Step Instructions:

1. Begin with 5 minutes of the Third Eye Sensing exercise.

2. Rub your palms together vigorously until they feel warm and energized.

3. Place your warm right palm over your third eye area (center of forehead), with your left palm over the back of your head.

4. Feel the energy flowing between your palms, through your head and third eye center.

5. Maintain this position for 2-3 minutes, breathing deeply and focusing on the sensations.

6. Remove your hands and return to a meditation posture.

7. Visualize a violet or indigo light at your third eye center, pulsing gently with each breath.

8. With each inhalation, imagine this light growing slightly brighter.

9. With each exhalation, imagine the light expanding slightly outward.

10. Continue for 10-15 minutes, then allow the visualization to fade and rest in simple awareness before concluding.

Integration Practice: Unifying the Three Techniques

The most profound benefits come from integrating these practices into a cohesive cultivation system. This final exercise combines elements from all three techniques into a single, powerful practice for awakening the upper dantian.

Exercise: Complete Upper Dantian Cultivation

Step-by-Step Instructions:

1. Begin with 5 minutes of Shen breathing to establish a foundation of clear energy.

2. Transition to Inner Light meditation, allowing natural luminosity to appear at your third eye center.

3. As the Inner Light stabilizes, begin to synchronize it with your breath—brightening slightly on inhalation, expanding on exhalation.

4. After 5-10 minutes, introduce the Third Eye Sensing technique, feeling an opening or awakening at the center of your forehead.

5. Maintain awareness of all three elements simultaneously: the breath moving Shen energy, the Inner Light illuminating, and the Third Eye center awakening.

6. Allow these three aspects to harmonize and unify, creating a singular experience of upper dantian activation.

7. Rest in this unified state for 10-15 minutes.

8. To conclude, gradually release all techniques and rest in simple, open awareness.

9. Take three deep breaths, feeling gratitude for your practice.

10. Slowly open your eyes, maintaining a subtle awareness of your awakened upper dantian as you return to normal activities.

Practice Guidelines

1. Consistency over intensity: Practice these techniques for shorter periods (15-20 minutes) daily rather than longer sessions less frequently.

2. Gentle attention: Never strain or force these practices. Maintaining a gentle, receptive awareness yields better results than aggressive effort.

3. Progressive development: Begin with the first exercise in each section, mastering it before moving to more advanced practices.

4. Integration with daily life: Throughout your day, occasionally bring awareness to your upper dantian, reconnecting with the sensations and qualities you experienced in formal practice.

5. Journal your experiences: Keep a record of sensations, insights, and changes you notice, both during practice and in daily life.

By dedicated practice of these techniques, you will gradually awaken the upper dantian, cultivating spiritual awareness, intuitive wisdom, and expanded consciousness. This awakening represents an important stage in the journey of inner cultivation, opening doorways to more refined states of being and perception.

AWAKENING THE UPPER DANTIAN

Practice Workbook & Journal

Welcome to your personal practice companion for the journey of awakening the upper dantian. This workbook is designed to guide your daily practice, track your progress, and deepen your understanding of the subtle energies of the upper center.

True mastery comes through consistent practice and mindful attention. Use this workbook to establish a regular routine, record your experiences, and witness your own evolution as you cultivate the spiritual awareness associated with the upper dantian.

Remember that this journey unfolds at its own pace. Some days may bring profound experiences, while others might seem ordinary. All are valuable parts of the path.

SECTION 1: PRACTICE SCHEDULE

7-Day Practice Plan

Day	Morning Practice (15-20 min)	Evening Practice (15-20 min)
1	Inner Light Meditation (Exercise 1)	Gentle breath awareness
2	Inner Light Meditation (Exercise 1)	Shen Breathing (Exercise 1)
3	Inner Light Meditation (Exercise 2)	Shen Breathing (Exercise 1)
4	Shen Breathing (Exercise 2)	Third Eye Sensing (Exercise 1)
5	Third Eye Sensing (Exercise 1)	Third Eye Energy Cultivation (Exercise 2)
6	Combined practice (5 min each)	Free choice of favorite technique

Day	Morning Practice (15-20 min)	Evening Practice (15-20 min)
7	Integration Practice (Complete Upper Dantian Cultivation)	Reflection and journaling

28-Day Advanced Practice Plan

Week 1: Foundation Building

- Focus on mastering the first exercise of each practice
- 15 minutes daily, alternating techniques
- Journal after each session

Week 2: Deepening Practice

- Introduce the second exercises
- Extend practice to 20 minutes daily
- Begin noticing effects throughout your day

Week 3: Integration

- Begin combining techniques
- Practice the Integration Exercise every other day
- Note any dreams or intuitive experiences in your journal

Week 4: Refinement

- Focus on subtlety and sensitivity
- Practice the complete Integration Exercise daily
- Record insights about your progress over the month

SECTION 2: PRACTICE TRACKING

Daily Practice Log

Date: _____

Practice completed:

- [ ] Inner Light Meditation - Ex. 1
- [ ] Inner Light Meditation - Ex. 2
- [ ] Shen Breathing - Ex. 1
- [ ] Shen Breathing - Ex. 2
- [ ] Third Eye Sensing - Ex. 1
- [ ] Third Eye Energy Cultivation - Ex. 2
- [ ] Integration Practice

Duration: _____ minutes

Time of day: □ Morning □ Afternoon □ Evening

Location: _____

Before practice:

- Physical sensations: _____
- Emotional state: _____
- Mental clarity (1-10): _____

During practice:

- Ease of concentration (1-10): _____
- Sensations observed: _____
- Challenges encountered: _____
- Insights or experiences: _____

After practice:

- Changes in physical sensations: _____
- Changes in emotional state: _____
- Changes in mental clarity (1-10): _____
- Overall quality of practice (1-10): _____

Notes for next practice: _____

SECTION 3: UPPER DANTIAN AWARENESS JOURNAL

Inner Light Meditation Reflections

Date: _____

What subtle sensations did you notice at your third eye center?

Describe any light, colors, or patterns you observed:

How did the quality of light change throughout your practice?

What helped you maintain focus on the Inner Light?

Insights or questions that arose during practice:

Shen Breathing Reflections

Date: _____

How did your breath quality change during the practice?

Describe the movement of energy you experienced:

How did synchronizing breath with awareness affect your experience?

Did you notice any connection between different energy centers?

Changes in your sense of self or consciousness during practice:

Third Eye Activation Reflections

Date: _____

Sensations experienced at the third eye center:

Quality of awareness when focusing on the third eye:

Any intuitive impressions or insights received:

Changes in perception during or after practice:

Questions or curiosities that arose during practice:

SECTION 4: WEEKLY REFLECTION

Week ending: _____

Overall consistency of practice this week: □ Excellent □ Good □ Fair □ Inconsistent

Most significant experiences or insights:

Most challenging aspects of practice:

Changes noticed in daily life:

- Physical: _____

- Emotional: _____
- Mental: _____
- Spiritual/Intuitive: _____

Questions that have arisen:

Adjustments needed for next week's practice:

Goals for the coming week:

SECTION 5: DEEPENING UNDERSTANDING

Upper Dantian Contemplation Questions

Take time to reflect on these questions, either in writing or meditation:

1. How would you describe the quality of consciousness associated with your upper dantian?
2. In what ways has your perception changed since beginning these practices?
3. What is the relationship between the light you perceive in meditation and your everyday awareness?
4. How does the upper dantian connect with the middle and lower centers in your experience?
5. What intuitive faculties have you noticed developing through these practices?

Self-Assessment: Mapping Your Progress

Rate your current experience (1-10):

Inner Light Perception

- Ability to perceive subtle light: _____
- Stability of the light once perceived: _____
- Clarity of the light quality: _____
- Integration of light awareness in daily life: _____

Breath-Spirit Connection

- Synchronization of breath and awareness: _____
- Sensing energy movement with breath: _____
- Refinement of breath quality: _____
- Ability to direct energy with breath: _____

Third Eye Activation

- Sensitivity at third eye center: _____
- Clarity of third eye perception: _____
- Integration of intuitive insights: _____
- Expansion of awareness beyond ordinary senses: _____

SECTION 6: SPECIAL EXPERIENCES LOG

Use this section to record particularly notable experiences during your practice or in daily life that may relate to upper dantian awakening.

Date: _____

Description of experience:

Context (during practice, dream, daily activity, etc.):

Insights gained from this experience:

Questions that arose from this experience:

SECTION 7: PRACTICE REFINEMENT NOTES

Inner Light Meditation Adjustments

Things that enhance my practice:

Posture adjustments that help:

Best time of day for this practice:

Shen Breathing Refinements

Breath rhythm that works best:

Visualizations that enhance energy flow:

Ways to deepen the breath-spirit connection:

Third Eye Activation Techniques

Most effective preparation methods:

Sensations that indicate activation:

Methods for maintaining third eye awareness:

SECTION 8: INTEGRATION WITH DAILY LIFE

Mindfulness Reminders

List 3-5 daily activities during which you can practice brief moments of upper dantian awareness:

1.
2.
3.
4.
5.

Intuitive Development Exercises

Record instances when you consciously used your intuition and the outcomes:

Date: _____

Situation requiring intuitive guidance:

How you accessed your intuition:

Guidance received:

Results of following (or not following) this guidance:

SECTION 9: MONTHLY REVIEW

Month: _____

Total practice sessions completed: _____

Most significant breakthroughs or insights:

Most notable changes in:

- Physical well-being: _____
- Emotional balance: _____
- Mental clarity: _____
- Intuitive capacity: _____
- Spiritual awareness: _____

Practices that were most beneficial:

Practices that were most challenging:

Questions for further exploration:

Goals for next month:

SECTION 10: PERSONAL NOTES AND INSIGHTS

Use this space for additional reflections, insights, questions, or experiences that don't fit elsewhere in the journal.

Remember that the journey of awakening the upper dantian is both profound and subtle. Progress may not always be linear, and experiences will vary from day to day. What matters most is your sincere and consistent practice.

As you continue working with these practices, maintain an attitude of curious exploration rather than forced achievement. The upper dantian responds best to gentle, persistent attention rather than aggressive effort.

May your practice bring you clarity, insight, and expanded awareness.

"The light of spirit resides within, waiting only for the gentle touch of your attention to reveal its luminous presence."

In our journey toward deeper self-understanding and spiritual growth, we arrive at a pivotal crossroads: the cultivation of presence and perception. This chapter explores three interconnected dimensions of consciousness that transcend ordinary awareness—non-dual awareness, observing the observer, and heart-mind alignment (Xin). These practices represent pathways to experience reality beyond our habitual, divided perception.

The modern world encourages constant distraction, analytical thinking, and separation. We often live divided lives—mind separated from body, self from others, thinking from feeling. This fragmentation creates suffering and prevents us from experiencing the wholeness that lies at our core. The practices in this chapter offer a remedy to this division, inviting us to discover a more integrated way of being.

As we explore these concepts, remember that they point to direct experiences rather than intellectual ideas. The true value comes from practice, not theory. The exercises provided are designed as experiential gateways—opportunities to taste these states firsthand rather than merely understand them conceptually.

Let us begin this exploration with openness and curiosity, recognizing that these practices have transformed lives across cultures and throughout history.

Non-Dual Awareness

Understanding Non-Duality

Non-dual awareness represents a fundamental shift in perception—moving beyond the subject-object divide that characterizes our ordinary consciousness. In conventional awareness, we experience ourselves as separate observers of an external world. We are "here" looking at objects that are "there." This dualistic perception creates a persistent sense of separation between self and other, observer and observed.

Non-dual awareness dissolves this boundary. It is a state where the perceived separation between the observer and the observed falls away, revealing a unified field of experience. This is not merely a philosophical concept but a direct experiential reality that traditions worldwide have recognized:

- In Buddhism, it relates to concepts like emptiness (śūnyatā) and the interdependent nature of all phenomena
- In Advaita Vedanta, it's expressed as the unity of Atman (individual consciousness) and Brahman (universal consciousness)
- In Taoism, it manifests as the harmonious flow with the Tao
- In contemplative Christian traditions, it appears as unitive consciousness or "the cloud of unknowing"

In non-dual awareness, we don't lose our ability to function or distinguish between objects. Rather, we recognize that these distinctions exist within a more fundamental unity. The ocean produces countless waves, each appearing unique, yet all are fundamentally water. Similarly, non-dual awareness recognizes the diversity of experience while perceiving its underlying unity.

Key Characteristics of Non-Dual Awareness

1. **Seamlessness**: Boundaries between self and world, inside and outside, become permeable and transparent.
2. **Immediacy**: Experience is direct, without the usual filter of conceptual thinking inserting itself between perceiver and perceived.
3. **Wholeness**: There's a sense of completeness rather than fragmentation—reality experienced as an integrated whole rather than isolated parts.
4. **Naturalness**: Non-dual awareness feels like returning home to our natural state rather than achieving something new.
5. **Timelessness**: The usual sense of time passing can dissolve into an expanded present moment.

Exercises for Cultivating Non-Dual Awareness

Exercise 1: The Seamless Field of Sound

Purpose: To experience non-separation between awareness and auditory experience.

Steps:

1. Find a quiet place to sit comfortably, either on a chair or cushion, with your spine naturally erect.
2. Close your eyes and take three deep breaths, allowing your body to settle.
3. Begin to notice the sounds in your environment. Don't try to identify or label them—simply let them be as they are.

4. Notice how we typically create a sense of separation: "I am here, hearing sounds out there." Feel this sense of separation.
5. Now, shift your attention to the awareness itself—the knowing of sound rather than the sounds as objects.
6. Ask yourself: "Where does my hearing end and the sound begin?" Rest in the space where this question leads.
7. Allow the distinction between "hearing" and "sound" to dissolve. Experience sounds not as objects you're perceiving but as events arising in awareness itself.
8. Notice how sounds simply emerge in consciousness without effort, already complete, requiring no "hearer" to make them real.
9. Expand this field of awareness to include all sounds, near and far, as one seamless field of experience.
10. Rest in this non-dual awareness of sound for 10-15 minutes.

Reflection Questions:

- What happens to your sense of being a separate "hearer" when you rest in this way?
- How does this experience differ from your usual way of listening?
- Do you notice any moments where the boundary between "you" and "sound" seems to dissolve?

Exercise 2: The Transparent Body

Purpose: To experience the body beyond the subject-object divide.

Steps:

1. Sit or lie down in a comfortable position where you can remain alert yet relaxed.
2. Close your eyes and allow your attention to settle into your body.
3. Notice how we typically experience the body as an object—something we have or possess rather than what we are.
4. Begin to scan through your body, starting from your feet and moving upward.
5. As you bring awareness to each area, drop the conceptual label (foot, leg, etc.) and experience the raw sensations directly—tingling, pressure, warmth, pulsing.

6. Instead of thinking "I am feeling sensations in my hand," simply be the experiencing of these sensations as they arise.
7. Ask yourself: "Who or what is aware of these sensations?" Don't answer intellectually—let the question open a space of direct knowing.
8. Allow the sense of a "body observer" separate from "body sensations" to relax and dissolve.
9. Experience your entire body as a field of sensation appearing in awareness, without center or periphery.
10. Rest in this transparent, boundaryless experience of embodiment for 15-20 minutes.

Reflection Questions:

- What happens to your usual sense of having a body when you practice this way?
- Did you notice any moments where the sensations weren't happening "to you" but simply occurring as awareness itself?
- How does this experience compare to your habitual way of relating to your body?

Exercise 3: Gazing Without Boundaries

Purpose: To experience visual perception beyond subject-object duality.

Steps:

1. Find a place where you can sit comfortably, facing an open space—perhaps a landscape, sky, or even a wall.
2. Sit with your eyes open, gazing softly without focusing on any particular object.
3. Notice your habitual way of seeing—identifying distinct objects separated from you as the viewer.
4. Now, gradually expand your field of vision to take in the entire visual field at once, including the peripheral areas.
5. Relax the eyes, softening your gaze so you're not focusing sharply on anything in particular.
6. Let go of naming or categorizing what you see. Experience colors, shapes, and movements directly, prior to conceptual labeling.
7. Feel into the space between you and what you're seeing. Is there really a boundary where "you" end and the "seen world" begins?

8. Allow the sense of being a "seer" separate from the "seen" to relax. Experience seeing happening by itself, not done by a separate self.
9. Rest in this boundaryless visual field, where perception happens without a perceiver, for 10-15 minutes.
10. When ready, gently return to normal perception while retaining a sense of the openness you've experienced.

Reflection Questions:

- What happens to your sense of being a separate observer when vision is experienced this way?
- Did you notice any shifts in your experience of space or boundaries?
- How does this way of seeing affect your sense of connection with your environment?

Observing the Observer

The Paradox of Self-Observation

Who is it that knows your experience? When you have a thought, who is aware of that thought? When an emotion arises, who notices it? The conventional answer is "I am"—but this raises a profound question: Who or what is this "I" that observes?

When we attempt to find this observer—this "I" that seems to be at the center of our experience—we encounter a fascinating paradox. Every time we try to observe the observer, what we find are only more objects of awareness: thoughts, sensations, images, feelings. The observer itself seems to perpetually recede from view, like an eye trying to see itself.

This leads to a revolutionary insight: perhaps the observer—the pure awareness at our core—cannot be found as an object because it is the very subject of all experience. It is not a thing to be observed but the observing itself. Not an entity within consciousness, but the consciousness within which all entities appear.

The Witness Consciousness

Spiritual traditions have long recognized this pure awareness as "witness consciousness" (sākṣī in Sanskrit) or "the observing self." This witnessing capacity:

- Is present throughout all states of consciousness (waking, dreaming, deep sleep)
- Remains unchanged while thoughts, emotions, and sensations constantly change
- Has no form or content of its own, yet illuminates all forms and contents
- Cannot be grasped conceptually but can be directly recognized

Cultivating familiarity with witness consciousness creates a profound shift in our relationship with experience. Rather than being completely identified with and overwhelmed by thoughts and emotions, we develop the capacity to be present with them from a space of openness and clarity.

Exercises for Observing the Observer

Exercise 1: The Source of Attention

Purpose: To trace attention back to its source.

Steps:

1. Sit comfortably in a quiet space where you won't be disturbed. Establish a posture that is alert yet relaxed.
2. Close your eyes and take several deep breaths, allowing your body and mind to settle.
3. Begin by noticing an external sound. Be aware that you are hearing it.
4. Now, shift your attention to a bodily sensation. Notice that the same awareness that knew the sound now knows this sensation.
5. Next, notice a thought or mental image arising. Observe that the same awareness that knew the sensation now knows this thought.
6. Continue shifting attention between different objects of awareness—sounds, sensations, thoughts, emotions—recognizing that the same knowing presence is aware of each.
7. Now ask: "Who or what is aware of all these experiences?" Don't answer conceptually—simply rest in the questioning itself.
8. Turn your attention around to look for this aware presence. Notice what happens when attention tries to find its own source.
9. Rest in the recognition that awareness itself cannot be found as an object, yet it is undeniably present as the knowing of all experience.
10. Remain in this recognition for 15-20 minutes, continually relaxing backward into the source of awareness itself.

Reflection Questions:

- What happens when you try to find the one who is aware?
- How does this practice affect your identification with thoughts and emotions?
- What qualities do you notice in the aware presence itself?

Exercise 2: Awareness Without Content

Purpose: To recognize awareness independent of its contents.

Steps:

1. Find a quiet place to practice without distractions. Sit in a comfortable, upright position.
2. Close your eyes and allow your mind to settle naturally without forcing stillness.
3. Notice the various contents of consciousness arising—thoughts, sensations, sounds, feelings—without getting involved in their stories.
4. As you notice each content, silently note: "This is an object of awareness, not awareness itself."
5. Begin to get curious about the awareness in which all these experiences are appearing. What is the nature of this knowing presence?
6. Whenever you notice yourself getting caught in thought, gently recognize: "Even this thought is appearing in awareness."
7. As the mind naturally cycles through periods of activity and quiet, notice that awareness itself remains constant throughout.
8. When the mind becomes very quiet, pay attention to the aware space in which silence is known. What qualities does this awareness have?
9. Rest in the recognition of awareness itself—not as a concept or object, but as the ever-present ground of all experience.
10. Continue this practice for 20-30 minutes, repeatedly relaxing back into awareness itself rather than following its contents.

Reflection Questions:

- Is awareness itself changeable, or only its contents?
- Can you recognize awareness even when thinking is active?
- How does resting as awareness rather than following thoughts change your experience?

Exercise 3: The Mirror and Reflections Practice

Purpose: To distinguish between awareness itself and its contents using the metaphor of a mirror and its reflections.

Steps:

1. Sit comfortably with your spine naturally erect. Take a few deep breaths to center yourself.
2. Imagine consciousness as a clear, pristine mirror. All experiences—thoughts, sensations, emotions, perceptions—are like reflections appearing in this mirror.
3. Begin to notice the current contents of your experience—sounds, bodily sensations, thoughts—and recognize each as a "reflection" in the mirror of awareness.
4. Notice how reflections continuously change—appearing, changing, disappearing—while the mirror itself remains unchanged.
5. When a thought arises, recognize: "This thought is a reflection in the mirror of awareness, not the mirror itself."
6. When an emotion arises, recognize: "This emotion is a reflection in the mirror of awareness, not the mirror itself."
7. Continue with all experiences, recognizing each as a temporary reflection distinct from the unchanging mirror.
8. Ask yourself: "Can a reflection ever damage or alter the mirror itself?" Feel how awareness remains untouched by its contents.
9. Gradually shift your identification from the reflections to the mirror itself. Rest as the aware space in which all experiences appear.
10. Remain in this practice for 15-20 minutes, continually recognizing the distinction between awareness and its contents.

Reflection Questions:

- How does identifying with the mirror rather than the reflections change your relationship with difficult thoughts or emotions?
- Can you find any experience that exists outside the mirror of awareness?
- What qualities do you notice in the mirror itself, independent of any particular reflection?

The Unified Heart-Mind

In Chinese contemplative traditions, particularly Confucianism, Taoism, and Chan Buddhism, the concept of Xin (心) holds profound significance. Often translated as "heart-mind," Xin represents the natural unity of what Western thinking typically divides into separate faculties of emotion and cognition, feeling and thinking.

The Chinese character 心 (xin) depicts the heart organ, reflecting the traditional understanding that the heart—not the brain—was the seat of both thinking and feeling. This wasn't merely a physical misattribution but a profound intuition that our cognitive and emotional lives are fundamentally unified at their source.

When heart and mind are aligned (Xin), we experience:

- Clarity without coldness
- Warmth without confusion
- Wisdom infused with compassion
- Understanding that is both cognitive and felt
- Action that emerges from both insight and care

The disintegration of Xin—the separation of heart from mind—creates numerous problems in our lives. When thinking operates divorced from feeling, it becomes dry, abstract, and potentially harmful. When feeling operates without clarity, it becomes overwhelming, confused, and reactive. Reunifying heart and mind returns us to our natural wholeness.

The Path to Heart-Mind Alignment

Cultivating Xin involves practices that bridge the artificial divide between cognitive and emotional aspects of our being. This integration happens at multiple levels:

1. **Physical**: Recognizing and releasing tensions that maintain the separation between head and heart in our bodies.
2. **Emotional**: Bringing clear awareness to our feeling states without either suppressing them or being overwhelmed by them.
3. **Cognitive**: Infusing our thinking with the qualities of heart—warmth, openness, and compassion.

4. **Energetic**: Cultivating a felt sense of connection between the head and heart centers in our subtle body.
5. **Contemplative**: Recognizing that pure awareness (observer) and loving presence (heart) are ultimately the same reality experienced in different ways.

The practices below are designed to cultivate these different dimensions of integration, gradually restoring the natural unified functioning of Xin.

Exercises for Heart-Mind Alignment (Xin)

Exercise 1: The Thread of Breath

Purpose: To establish an energetic and attentional connection between head and heart centers.

Steps:

1. Sit comfortably with your spine naturally erect. Place one hand on your heart center in the middle of your chest.
2. Take several deep, slow breaths, allowing your body to relax and your attention to settle.
3. Bring awareness to your head—the location of thinking, perceiving, and analyzing. Notice any sensations in this area.
4. Now, bring awareness to your heart center in the middle of your chest. Notice any sensations in this area.
5. Imagine your breath as a luminous thread connecting these two centers. As you inhale, feel the breath energy flowing from your heart to your head.
6. As you exhale, feel the breath energy flowing from your head back to your heart.
7. Continue this circular breathing pattern, creating a continuous flow between head and heart.
8. As you practice, silently repeat with each breath cycle: "Thinking and feeling unified... clarity and warmth as one."
9. Notice any sense of increased coherence, harmony, or unity between cognitive and emotional aspects of your experience.
10. Continue this practice for 10-15 minutes, gradually allowing the distinction between head and heart centers to soften.

Reflection Questions:

- How does your thinking change when connected more directly with your heart center?
- What qualities do you notice in your awareness when head and heart are linked?
- Where in your life do you experience heart and mind operating separately, and how might this practice help?

Exercise 2: Cognitive-Emotional Integration

Purpose: To bring together cognitive understanding and emotional intelligence when facing situations.

Steps:

1. Find a quiet space where you can reflect undisturbed. Have a journal ready for notes.
2. Think of a current situation in your life that requires both understanding and care—perhaps a relationship challenge, a decision, or a creative project.
3. First, approach this situation from a purely cognitive perspective. Ask yourself:
   - What are the facts and details I know about this situation?
   - What logical analysis can I apply here?
   - What solutions seem rational from this perspective? Write down your thoughts.
4. Notice the quality of this thinking. Is it clear but perhaps cold? Precise but maybe lacking depth?
5. Now, approach the same situation from a purely emotional perspective. Ask yourself:
   - What feelings arise when I consider this situation?
   - What do I care about most deeply here?
   - What response feels most caring or compassionate? Write down these reflections.
6. Notice the quality of this emotional approach. Is it warm but perhaps lacking clarity? Connected but maybe not strategic?
7. Now, place one hand on your heart and one on your forehead. Take several deep breaths, connecting these centers.
8. From this unified heart-mind space, approach the situation again, asking:
   - What understanding emerges when my thinking is warmed by my heart?
   - What clarity comes to my emotions when illuminated by my mind?

- What response honors both wisdom and compassion? Write down what emerges.
9. Notice the different quality of this integrated perspective. How does it compare to either perspective alone?
10. Consider how you might apply this integrated heart-mind wisdom to the actual situation in your life.

Reflection Questions:

- How does your understanding of the situation differ when approached from the unified heart-mind?
- What new possibilities become visible that weren't apparent from either perspective alone?
- How might this practice help you navigate complex situations in your daily life?

Exercise 3: The Compassionate Observer

Purpose: To integrate the witnessing quality of pure awareness with the warmth and care of the heart.

Steps:

1. Sit comfortably in a quiet place where you won't be disturbed. Establish a posture that is both dignified and relaxed.
2. Begin by connecting with the witnessing quality of consciousness—the clear, spacious awareness that observes without judgment.
3. Notice thoughts, sensations, and emotions arising, simply witnessing them without becoming involved in their content.
4. After establishing this witnessing presence, bring attention to your heart center. Feel or imagine a warm glow of compassionate awareness in this area.
5. Allow this heart-centered warmth to gradually permeate your witnessing presence, infusing the clear observer with qualities of kindness and care.
6. When challenging thoughts or emotions arise, meet them with this compassionate awareness—clear seeing combined with warm acceptance.
7. Notice how this compassionate observer relates differently to experience than either cold observation or emotional reactivity would.
8. Continue alternating between emphasizing the clear seeing quality and the warm heart quality, gradually allowing them to interpenetrate and unify.

9. Rest in this integrated awareness that is simultaneously crystal clear and warmly present, witnessing all experience with compassionate clarity.
10. Practice this for 20-30 minutes, noticing how this unified heart-mind awareness (Xin) relates to whatever arises in your experience.

Reflection Questions:

- How does compassionate observation differ from either detached witnessing or emotional involvement?
- What happens to difficult thoughts or emotions when met with this unified heart-mind awareness?
- How might cultivating this compassionate observer affect your relationships with others and yourself?

Integration of the Three Practices

The three dimensions explored in this chapter—non-dual awareness, observing the observer, and heart-mind alignment (Xin)—are not separate practices but complementary facets of a unified approach to awakened consciousness.

Non-dual awareness reveals the fundamental unity of subject and object, dissolving the sense of separation that creates suffering. Observing the observer points us to the true nature of awareness itself—the ground of all experience that cannot be found as an object. Heart-mind alignment (Xin) integrates the clarity of witnessing with the warmth of compassion, creating a unified response to life that is both wise and loving.

Together, these practices form a complete approach to transformation:

- Non-dual awareness liberates us from the illusion of separation
- Observing the observer reveals our true identity as awareness itself
- Heart-mind alignment infuses this recognition with compassionate presence

The ultimate goal is not to perfect any single practice but to allow their insights to interpenetrate and transform our entire being—leading to a life characterized by clear seeing, open-hearted presence, and spontaneous appropriate action.

Living from Presence

As these practices mature, they gradually infuse our everyday lives. What begins as formal meditation becomes a natural way of being. We find ourselves responding to situations with greater spontaneity, wisdom, and care.

The boundaries between meditation and daily life begin to dissolve. We discover that presence isn't something we do but what we fundamentally are. Each moment becomes an opportunity to recognize and live from this truth—whether we're engaged in deep contemplation, meaningful work, or washing the dishes.

The journey of cultivating presence and perception doesn't lead to a fixed destination but to an ever-deepening embodiment of our true nature. It's a continuous unfolding that reveals increasing degrees of freedom, clarity, and compassionate engagement with all of life.

As you continue working with these practices, be patient with yourself. Progress isn't linear, and insights often come unexpectedly. Trust the process and remember that each moment of genuine presence—even briefly glimpsed—is complete in itself and gradually transforms your entire way of being in the world.

Further Reading and Resources

For those wishing to explore these practices more deeply, the following resources are recommended:

Non-Dual Awareness

- "The Transparency of Things" by Rupert Spira
- "Awakening to the Dream" by Leo Hartong
- "The Experience of No-Self" by Bernadette Roberts
- "I Am That" by Nisargadatta Maharaj

Observing the Observer

- "The Untethered Soul" by Michael Singer
- "Awareness" by Anthony De Mello
- "Shift Into Freedom" by Loch Kelly
- "The Attention Revolution" by Alan Wallace

Heart-Mind Alignment (Xin)

- "Cultivating the Empty Field" translated by Dan Leighton
- "A New Earth" by Eckhart Tolle
- "True Love" by Thich Nhat Hanh
- "Anam Cara" by John O'Donohue

May your journey into these practices bring increasing clarity, peace, and compassionate presence to your life and to all those you encounter.

Workbook: Cultivating Presence and Perception

Journal Reflections

1. How does your perception of self and other shift during non-dual awareness practices?

_____

2. What insights have you gained through observing the observer? Has it changed how you relate to thoughts or emotions?

_____

3. In what ways do you experience alignment or misalignment between heart and mind in daily life?

_____

4. How does compassionate witnessing affect your ability to be present with yourself and others?

_____

5. Which practice in this chapter resonated most deeply with you, and why?

_____

Practice Tracker: Presence and Perception

Use this table to track your practices over the week.

Date	Practice	Duration (min)	Noted Experiences	Emotional/Mental State After

Non-Dual Awareness Log

Note your direct experiences of non-dual awareness. What shifted? Did any boundaries dissolve?

_____
_____
_____

Observer Awareness Log

Describe your experiences when observing the observer. What emerged when trying to find the one who is aware?

_____
_____
_____

Heart-Mind Alignment Log

Reflect on moments of heart-mind integration. How did this affect your clarity, emotional balance, and insight?

_____
_____
_____

Dreams have been regarded as sacred messengers across cultures and throughout time. From the dream temples of ancient Greece to the vision quests of indigenous peoples, humans have sought wisdom, healing, and spiritual connection through their nighttime experiences. This chapter explores three powerful approaches to working with dreams as a spiritual practice: dream journaling and lucid dreaming, intention and symbolic vision, and the Eastern practice of Nighttime Shen Gong.

Dream Journaling and Lucid Dreaming

The Sacred Act of Recording Dreams

Dream journaling is more than simply writing down what you remember upon waking—it is an invitation to the unconscious, a declaration that you value the messages from your deeper self. When we commit to recording our dreams, we strengthen the connection between our conscious and unconscious minds, gradually building a bridge that allows more information to flow between these realms.

The ancient Egyptians believed dreams were messages from the gods, while Aboriginal Australians saw dreamtime as the foundation of reality itself. Modern psychological perspectives recognize dreams as windows into our unconscious processes, but many spiritual traditions go further, suggesting dreams can provide access to collective wisdom, ancestral knowledge, and even prophetic insight.

Dreams speak primarily through symbols and emotions rather than linear thought. A river in your dream may represent the flow of life, a transitional period, or the boundary between conscious and unconscious. A house might symbolize your psyche, with different rooms representing aspects of yourself. By recording and reflecting on these symbols consistently, you develop personal dream literacy—an understanding of your unique symbolic language.

Lucid Dreaming as Spiritual Practice

Lucid dreaming—becoming aware that you are dreaming while remaining in the dream state—opens extraordinary possibilities for spiritual exploration. When lucid, you can consciously interact with dream figures, ask questions of your unconscious, practice spiritual exercises, or simply witness the dream with full awareness.

Tibetan Buddhist dream yoga and various shamanic traditions have long utilized lucid dreaming as a spiritual technology. These practices recognize that the lucid dream state offers a unique opportunity to explore consciousness beyond ordinary waking reality. In this state, the constraints of physical laws are loosened, allowing for experiences that can profoundly shift our understanding of reality and ourselves.

The value of lucid dreaming lies not in controlling the dream for entertainment but in using this special state of consciousness for spiritual inquiry and growth. When we become lucid, we can practice presence, compassion, and non-attachment within the dream—skills that translate into our waking life. We can also use lucidity to heal emotional wounds by confronting and transforming dream scenarios that reflect our fears or unresolved issues.

Exercises for Dream Journaling and Lucid Dreaming

Exercise 1: Sacred Dream Journal Initiation

1. Obtain a journal dedicated solely to your dreams.
2. Before using it, hold the journal in your hands and set your intention aloud: "This journal is a sacred vessel for my dream experiences. As I record my dreams here, may I receive guidance, healing, and wisdom."
3. Place the journal and a pen beside your bed each night.
4. Upon waking—even from brief moments of consciousness during the night—immediately write down whatever dream fragments you recall, without censoring or analyzing.
5. Date each entry and note any significant life events or questions you had before sleep.
6. After recording the dream content, write about any emotions, sensations, or intuitive insights related to the dream.
7. At the end of each week, review your entries and look for patterns, recurring symbols, or themes.

Exercise 2: Reality Testing for Lucid Dreaming

1. Choose 3-5 "reality checks" from the following list:
   - Push your finger against your palm to see if it passes through

- Look at a digital clock or text, look away, then look back to see if it changes
- Try to breathe while pinching your nose
- Look at your hands and count your fingers
- Ask yourself, "Am I dreaming?" while genuinely considering the possibility

2. Perform these reality checks mindfully 10-15 times throughout your day, especially during events that commonly occur in your dreams.
3. As you perform each check, maintain a state of curiosity rather than automaticity. Truly question your reality in that moment.
4. Before sleep, affirm: "Tonight in my dreams, I will recognize when I am dreaming and become lucid."
5. When you achieve lucidity, resist the urge to control everything. Instead, practice being present with the dream, observing its nature with calm awareness.
6. Ask the dream or a dream figure, "What wisdom do you have for me?" or "What do I need to know right now?"
7. Record your experiences upon waking, noting both successful and unsuccessful attempts.

Exercise 3: Dream Incubation for Spiritual Guidance

1. Before sleep, identify a specific question or area where you seek guidance.
2. Write this question in your dream journal.
3. Create a simple ritual that signals to your unconscious that you're seeking dream guidance:
   - Light a candle (safely) and state your intention
   - Hold a symbolic object related to your question as you fall asleep
   - Repeat a phrase such as "Tonight, I will receive guidance about..."
4. As you drift toward sleep, visualize yourself receiving clear insights in your dreams.
5. Upon waking, immediately record any dreams, even if they don't seem obviously related to your question.
6. Look for symbolic or metaphorical answers rather than literal ones.
7. Practice this for seven consecutive nights, then review all dreams together for deeper patterns.

Intention and Symbolic Vision

The Power of Conscious Dreaming

While lucid dreaming occurs during sleep, symbolic vision practices help us access dream-like states while awake. These practices blur the boundary between waking and dreaming, revealing the continuous nature of consciousness across different states of being.

Throughout history, mystics, artists, and visionaries have cultivated the ability to enter visionary states that combine the logic of waking consciousness with the symbolic richness of dreams. The shamanic journey, active imagination (developed by Carl Jung), guided visualization, and contemplative prayer all represent different approaches to this territory.

At the heart of these practices is intention—the conscious direction of awareness toward specific purposes or questions. Unlike passive daydreaming, intentional symbolic vision requires both focus and receptivity, guiding attention while remaining open to what emerges from beyond the conscious mind.

Working with Personal and Universal Symbols

Symbolic vision draws upon both personal symbols (unique to your psyche) and archetypal symbols (shared across cultures). Your personal symbols gain power through your emotional connection to them, while archetypal symbols—like the tree of life, the wise elder, or the sacred mountain—carry collective psychic energy accumulated through countless human experiences.

By working with symbols intentionally, we develop a two-way relationship with our unconscious. We learn to speak its language while also bringing consciousness to aspects of ourselves that typically operate below awareness. This dialogue between conscious and unconscious creates an integrated wisdom greater than either alone could produce.

Symbolic vision allows us to re-enchant our relationship with reality. The modern world often treats symbols as mere metaphors or psychological tools, but traditional wisdom understands symbols as gateways to dimensions of reality not accessible through ordinary perception. When we engage with symbols as living presences rather than mental constructs, we open ourselves to their transformative power.

Exercise 4: Sanctuary Creation

1. Find a quiet space where you won't be disturbed for at least 30 minutes.
2. Sit comfortably with your spine erect but not rigid.
3. Close your eyes and take seven deep breaths, releasing tension with each exhalation.
4. Visualize yourself walking along a path in nature that feels inviting.
5. As you walk, affirm: "I am now creating my inner sanctuary, a sacred space between worlds."
6. Allow the path to lead you to a clearing or special location that feels right to you.
7. Take time to develop this space in detail—notice the landscape, time of day, colors, sounds, and how it feels to be there.
8. Create a specific feature that will serve as your working space: perhaps a circle of stones, a small temple, a tree with roots forming a seat, or whatever resonates.
9. Declare this space sacred and protected, a meeting ground between your conscious and unconscious mind.
10. End your first visit by affirming you will return, then visualize yourself walking back along the path to ordinary awareness.
11. Record the details of your sanctuary in your journal, including a sketch if possible.
12. Return to this sanctuary whenever you practice symbolic vision work.

Exercise 5: Symbol Dialogue

1. In your sanctuary (created in Exercise 4), invite a symbol or figure to appear that represents a quality you wish to develop (wisdom, courage, compassion, etc.).
2. Allow the symbol to take form without controlling its appearance. It may manifest as a person, animal, plant, object, or something unexpected.
3. When the symbol appears, greet it respectfully and thank it for coming.
4. Ask the symbol three questions:
    - "What is your name or how would you like me to address you?"
    - "What quality or wisdom do you embody that I need right now?"
    - "Is there a message or practice you wish to share with me?"
5. Listen with your inner senses—you might hear words, see images, or simply know the answers intuitively.

6. If appropriate, ask if there is a way you can honor this symbol in your daily life.
7. Thank the symbol and end the dialogue.
8. Return to normal awareness and immediately record the experience.
9. Look for ways to integrate the symbol's wisdom through a daily practice or reminder.
10. Return to dialogue with this symbol regularly, developing the relationship over time.

Exercise 6: Symbolic Vision for Healing

1. After entering your sanctuary, bring to mind a situation in your life that feels unresolved or painful.
2. Without analyzing, allow this situation to take symbolic form in your inner vision.
3. Observe the symbol with compassionate awareness, noting its appearance, energy, and your emotional response.
4. Ask this symbol: "What do you represent in my life?"
5. Then ask: "How are you trying to help me, even though it may be causing pain?"
6. Listen deeply to the response, which may come in any sensory form.
7. Ask: "How might you be transformed in a way that serves my highest good?"
8. Allow the symbol to transform naturally, without forcing change. This transformation may be dramatic or subtle.
9. When the transformation feels complete, ask the new form: "What practice or understanding will help me integrate this healing?"
10. Thank the symbol and return to normal awareness.
11. Record your experience, then identify one concrete action you can take based on the insight received.
12. Repeat this process with the same issue weekly until resolution feels complete.

Nighttime Shen Gong

The Taoist Approach to Dream Cultivation

Nighttime Shen Gong represents a sophisticated approach to spiritual dreaming from the Taoist tradition. "Shen" refers to spirit or consciousness, while "Gong" means cultivation or practice. Unlike many Western approaches that focus on dream interpretation or lucidity, Nighttime Shen Gong emphasizes the cultivation of consciousness during the transition states between waking and sleeping.

Taoists understand that the boundary between sleeping and waking is not as rigid as we typically believe. The hypnagogic state (falling asleep) and hypnopompic state (waking up) are viewed as powerful gateways where the practitioner can maintain awareness while the body enters deep rest. In these liminal states, the spirit (Shen) can be nourished and developed through specific attention practices.

Traditional Chinese medicine recognizes that different organs and energy systems process and release different emotions during the night. By understanding this rhythm, practitioners can harmonize their consciousness with these natural cycles, facilitating emotional processing and spiritual growth during sleep.

The Three Treasures in Dream Practice

Taoist inner alchemy works with three treasures: Jing (essence), Qi (vital energy), and Shen (spirit). Nighttime Shen Gong focuses particularly on refining Qi into Shen during sleep, transforming physical and emotional energy into spiritual awareness.

Dreams are understood as the movement of Hun (ethereal soul) during sleep. The quality of this movement—and thus the nature of our dreams—depends on the balance of Yin and Yang energies within us and how well we've cultivated our Three Treasures during waking hours. Nighttime practices complement daytime cultivation, creating a continuous circuit of spiritual development.

Unlike approaches that seek to control dreams, Nighttime Shen Gong emphasizes aligning with natural processes. The practitioner learns to "set the field" before sleep through specific postures, breathing methods, and mental focuses that create optimal conditions for spiritual dreaming without imposing rigid expectations.

Exercises for Nighttime Shen Gong

Exercise 7: Evening Qi Washing

1. One hour before bedtime, reduce exposure to screens and stimulating activities.
2. Stand with feet shoulder-width apart, knees slightly bent.
3. Rub your hands together vigorously until they feel warm.

4. Place your palms over your face and imagine washing away the day's concerns with golden light.
5. Gently brush your hands from forehead to chin seven times, visualizing tension dissolving.
6. Place your left palm over your heart center and right palm over your lower abdomen (lower dantian).
7. Breathe naturally, imagining with each inhale that golden light collects in your lower dantian.
8. With each exhale, feel this light circulating up to your heart and throughout your body.
9. Continue for 5-10 minutes, allowing your breathing to become progressively deeper and slower.
10. Complete by gently rubbing both kidneys (lower back) with your palms for 36 circular motions.
11. This practice clears accumulated stress-energy that might otherwise process through disturbing dreams.

Exercise 8: Dream-Entry Posture and Breath

1. Lie on your right side with knees slightly bent.
2. Place your right hand under your right cheek or ear, and your left hand on your left thigh.
3. Arrange pillows for comfort while maintaining this position.
4. Close your eyes and bring attention to your breath.
5. Begin counting backwards from 100 with each exhale.
6. As you count, practice "spiraling breath":
   - Imagine your inhale moving down your spine to your tailbone
   - Your exhale spirals up the front of your torso to your head
7. Allow your counting to become increasingly hazy as you drift toward sleep.
8. Maintain the gentle intention: "I remain aware as my body sleeps."
9. If you notice you've lost count, simply resume from where you remember without judgment.
10. This practice creates a smooth transition of consciousness from waking to sleeping while maintaining a thread of awareness.

Exercise 9: Three-Cycle Dream Integration

1. Set your intention to wake briefly after each sleep cycle (approximately every 90 minutes).
2. Place your dream journal within easy reach.

3. When you naturally wake between cycles:
    o   Remain still with eyes closed
    o   Notice any dream fragments or energetic sensations
    o   Record brief notes without fully waking if possible
    o   If fully alert, practice the following before returning to sleep:
4. Place your tongue against the roof of your mouth.
5. Take three deep breaths, imagining gathering the essence of your dream experience.
6. Silently ask: "What wisdom does this dream contain?"
7. Allow an answer to form without analysis.
8. As you drift back to sleep, hold the intention: "I receive the teaching of this dream and move deeper."
9. Upon final waking, review all notes and write a complete entry integrating insights from all cycles.
10. Look for patterns across the different sleep cycles, which often reveal progression through different levels of processing.

Integration: The Continuous Journey

The practices in this chapter are not separate techniques but complementary approaches to the same territory—the rich landscape of consciousness that exists beyond ordinary waking awareness. Dream journaling helps you remember and value your dream experiences; lucid dreaming develops your capacity for awareness within dreams; symbolic vision brings dream-like wisdom into waking life; and Nighttime Shen Gong harmonizes your energy system to support spiritual dreaming.

As you work with these practices, you may notice that the boundaries between different states of consciousness gradually become more permeable. Dreams may become more vivid and meaningful, daily life may take on a more dreamlike quality, and you may discover a continuous thread of awareness that persists through waking, dreaming, and deep sleep.

This journey of inner exploration has no final destination. Each night offers a new opportunity to venture into the depths of consciousness, each dream contains potential insights, and each morning brings the sacred responsibility of integrating what you've discovered. Through consistent practice, you develop not only greater understanding of yourself but also a more intimate relationship with the mystery of existence itself.

Remember that spiritual dreaming is not about escaping ordinary reality but about recognizing the extraordinary dimensions that exist within and alongside it. By honoring your dreams as meaningful communications from deeper aspects of consciousness, you enrich your waking life and expand your understanding of what it means to be fully human.

Recommended Reading

1. **Dream Gates: A Journey into Active Dreaming** by Robert Moss
2. **Inner Work: Using Dreams and Active Imagination for Personal Growth** by Robert A. Johnson
3. **The Tibetan Yogas of Dream and Sleep** by Tenzin Wangyal Rinpoche
4. **Dreamgates: Exploring the Worlds of Soul, Imagination, and Life Beyond Death** by Robert Moss
5. **The Divinity Code to Understanding Your Dreams and Visions** by Adam Thompson and Adrian Beale
6. **Lucid Dreaming: Gateway to the Inner Self** by Robert Waggoner
7. **The Tao of Natural Breathing** by Dennis Lewis
8. **Awakening the Sacred Body** by Tenzin Wangyal Rinpoche
9. **The Secret of the Golden Flower: A Chinese Book of Life** translated by Richard Wilhelm
10. **Dreams of Light: The Profound Daytime Practice of Lucid Dreaming** by Andrew Holecek

Workbook: Spiritual Dreams and Inner Journeying

Part 1: Dream Journaling & Lucid Dreaming

Exercise 1: Sacred Dream Journal Initiation

Reflection Prompts:

- What was your intention when you began this dream journal?
- What emotions or images stood out in this week's dreams?
- Are there any recurring symbols or themes?

Weekly Review:

- Three symbols that appeared most often:
- Patterns I noticed:
- Insights or guidance I received:

Exercise 2: Reality Testing for Lucid Dreaming

Daily Tracker (7 Days)

Date Reality Checks Performed Lucid Dream? Notes/Reflections

Reflection Prompts:

- What triggers seemed to work best for initiating lucidity?
- How did it feel to be lucid in your dreams?
- What messages or guidance emerged during lucidity?

Exercise 3: Dream Incubation for Spiritual Guidance

Daily Practice Tracker (7 Days)

Date Incubation Question Symbol/Object Used Dream Received? Insights

Final Review:

- How did your dreams reflect your question?
- What symbolic responses stood out?
- What guidance do you feel you received?

Part 2: Intention & Symbolic Vision

Exercise 4: Sanctuary Creation

Journal Prompts:

- Describe your sanctuary in full detail:
- What sensations and emotions did you feel there?
- How did your body and energy respond to the space?

Sketch: *(Include a drawing or map of your sanctuary)*

Exercise 5: Symbol Dialogue

Session Log:

Date Symbol Encountered Messages Received Feeling After Session

Integration Reflection:

- How can I embody or honor this symbol in my daily life?
- What quality or wisdom did I most need?

Exercise 6: Symbolic Vision for Healing

Session Journal:

- What situation or issue did you bring into the session?
- What symbol appeared to represent this issue?
- How did it transform?
- What message did you receive for integration?
- What action will you take based on this experience?

Progress Tracker:

- How has your relationship with this issue changed over multiple sessions?

Part 3: Nighttime Shen Gong

Exercise 7: Evening Qi Washing

Nightly Tracker (7 Days)

Date Start Time Duration Physical Sensations Emotional Shift

Reflection Prompts:

- Did you notice a difference in dream quality after this practice?
- What energy or tension did you feel released?

Exercise 8: Dream-Entry Posture and Breath

Sleep Log (7 Days)

Date Able to Maintain Awareness? Dream Clarity Insights or Symbols

Reflection Prompts:

- Was it easier to fall asleep or stay aware?
- How did the breathwork influence your dream transitions?

Dream Integration Log (3 Days)

Cycle Dream Notes Emotional Quality Insights Gained

1

2

3

Post-Practice Reflection:

- What themes connected across sleep cycles?
- What overall message did you receive?

Final Integration & Reflections

Weekly Summary Prompts:

- How has your relationship with dreaming changed?
- What new insights have emerged about yourself?
- How do you feel more connected to your inner guidance?
- What practices will you continue, and how will you refine them?

Quote for Reflection:

"Each dream contains the seed of awakening. To honor your dreams is to listen to the deeper truth of your own soul."

PART IV: Internal Alchemy – Shen to Emptiness

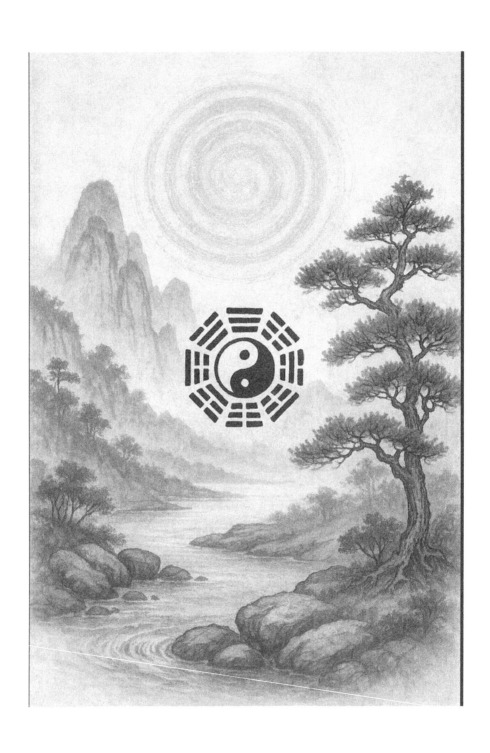

The Symbolic Language of Taoist Alchemy

Taoist inner alchemy, or neidan, represents one of humanity's most sophisticated systems for understanding and transforming consciousness. Unlike Western alchemy's focus on transmuting physical substances, Taoist alchemy operates primarily within the subtle energetic body, using richly symbolic language to describe internal processes of transformation.

At the heart of this tradition lies a complex symbolic language designed to both reveal and conceal. The Taoist alchemists employed imagery from metallurgy, pharmacology, astronomy, and nature to encode practices meant to refine and transmute the fundamental substances of life. Three primary symbols form the core vocabulary:

The cauldron (ding) represents the energetic centers of the body where transformation occurs—primarily the lower dantian (below the navel), middle dantian (at the heart), and upper dantian (between the eyebrows).

The furnace (lu) signifies the controlled internal heat that powers transformation, associated with specific breathing techniques and meditative focus.

The elixir (dan) denotes the refined essence that emerges through practice—the spiritual gold that confers longevity, wisdom, and ultimately, immortality.

These symbols operate within a comprehensive cosmology based on the interplay of yin and yang, the five elements (wood, fire, earth, metal, water), and the three treasures (jing/essence, qi/energy, shen/spirit). The language of inner alchemy deliberately parallels external processes: "lead" represents primordial, heavy energies that must be transmuted into the "gold" of refined consciousness.

Understanding this symbolic language requires recognizing its multi-layered nature. The texts speak simultaneously of physical processes (breathing, subtle sensations), energetic phenomena (movement of qi), and spiritual transformations (cultivation of consciousness). For the practitioner, these are not merely poetic metaphors but precise technical instructions for experiential exploration.

Fire and Water Phases

Within the laboratory of the body, the alchemical process unfolds through distinct phases involving the interplay of fire and water. These elements represent fundamental polarities within human experience: fire embodies yang qualities of heat, activity, and expansion, while water encompasses yin qualities of coolness, receptivity, and consolidation.

The fire and water phases of practice follow the natural cycles observed in the cosmos—daily, monthly, seasonal, and yearly rhythms that reflect the dance between these primordial forces. The classic description presents:

1. Kan (Water) and Li (Fire) - These trigrams from the *I Ching* represent primal cosmic forces that have become inverted in ordinary human experience. The practice aims to restore their proper relationship.

2. Lesser Water and Fire Phase - The initial stage focuses on gathering and circulating energy through the small heavenly orbit (microcosmic orbit), linking the governing and conception vessels along the spine and front of the body.

3. Greater Water and Fire Phase - The advanced practice extends to the greater heavenly orbit, incorporating the twelve primary meridians and transforming the three treasures.

4. Greatest Water and Fire Phase - The final refinement where fire and water achieve perfect balance, and yin and yang return to primordial unity.

The practice involves precise timing in accordance with natural cycles. Practitioners learn to recognize and harmonize with these rhythms—working with fire at certain times of day or seasons, and with water at others. This cyclical approach prevents extremes and maintains balance throughout the transformative journey.

Practically, the fire phase often involves active, warming practices that gather and direct energy, while the water phase emphasizes receptive, cooling practices that collect and preserve essence. The skilled practitioner learns to regulate these phases with increasing subtlety, creating the optimal conditions for transformation within the cauldron of the body.

Shen Fusion into Emptiness

The culmination of inner alchemical work involves the refinement and fusion of shen (spirit) into the state of emptiness (xu), a process that transcends dualistic consciousness and returns the practitioner to the primordial state of unity.

Shen represents the most refined aspect of the three treasures (jing, qi, and shen). While jing relates to physical essence and qi to vital energy, shen embodies spiritual consciousness—the illuminating principle within human awareness. In ordinary experience, shen remains fragmented and externally directed through the senses. The alchemical work aims to gather these scattered aspects of consciousness and return them to their source.

The process unfolds through several distinct stages:

1. Gathering Shen - Practitioners learn to withdraw consciousness from external fixations and collect it within. Meditation practices focus on "turning the light around" to illuminate the inner world rather than the outer.

2. Refining Shen - Through sustained attention, the quality of consciousness becomes increasingly clear, bright, and stable. This refinement purifies shen of habitual patterns and emotional distortions.

3. Fusing Shen - The various aspects of consciousness (associated with the five elements and corresponding emotions and organs) are harmonized and integrated into a unified field of awareness.

4. Shen Returning to Emptiness - In the final phase, even the subtlest sense of separate identity dissolves as shen merges with the boundless field of primordial emptiness—not a void, but the pregnant potential from which all phenomena arise.

This merging with emptiness represents not the extinction of consciousness but its ultimate fulfillment. The teachings describe this as "returning to the source," where the drop of individual awareness rejoins the ocean of universal consciousness. From this realization emerges the "immortal embryo" or "spirit body" (yangshen), a vehicle of pure consciousness no longer bound by the limitations of ordinary existence.

Practical Exercises

Exercise 1: Working with the Symbolic Language

Purpose: To develop intuitive understanding of alchemical symbolism.

Steps:

1. Set aside 20 minutes in a quiet space with a journal.

2. Choose one alchemical symbol (cauldron, furnace, lead, gold, etc.).

3. Close your eyes and visualize this symbol, allowing it to take form in your imagination.

4. Note any sensations, emotions, or insights that arise.

5. Open your eyes and write freely about what the symbol means to you on three levels:

   - Physical body and sensations

   - Energetic qualities and movements

   - Spiritual or consciousness significance

6. Compare your personal insights with traditional interpretations.

7. Repeat with a different symbol each day for one week.

Exercise 2: Balancing Fire and Water

Purpose: To experience and regulate the interplay of fire and water energies.

Steps:

1. Sit in a comfortable meditation posture with your spine upright.

2. Focus attention on your breath for 5 minutes, establishing calm awareness.

3. Bring attention to your kidneys region (lower back) and visualize cool, blue water essence gathering there.

4. Next, bring attention to your heart region and visualize warm, red fire essence gathering there.

5. Inhale and imagine water essence rising from kidneys to heart.

6. Exhale and imagine fire essence descending from heart to kidneys.

7. Continue this circulation for 10-15 minutes, noticing the qualities of each energy.

8. Observe the gradual harmonizing of these opposites as they meet and blend.

9. Complete by gathering the blended energy at your lower dantian (below navel).

10. Record your experiences, noting any imbalances between fire and water elements.

Exercise 3: Progressive Shen Refinement

Purpose: To experience the stages of gathering and refining spiritual consciousness.

Steps:

1. Find a quiet place where you won't be disturbed for 30 minutes.

2. Sit with eyes partially closed, gazing softly downward.

3. Gathering Phase (10 minutes):

   - Notice how your attention typically scatters through the five senses.

- Systematically withdraw attention from each sense: sounds, physical sensations, smells, tastes, and finally visual stimuli.

- Imagine collecting these streams of awareness like gathering scattered light into a single beam.

4. Refining Phase (10 minutes):

- Direct the gathered awareness to the space between your eyebrows.

- Visualize this awareness as a pearl of light, becoming increasingly clear and bright.

- When distractions arise, gently reabsorb them back into the pearl.

5. Fusing Phase (10 minutes):

- Allow the pearl of awareness to descend to your heart center.

- Feel it expanding outward while maintaining its clarity and brightness.

- Notice how this unified awareness embraces all experiences without becoming fragmented.

6. To conclude, rest in open awareness without effort or focus for 5 minutes.

7. Journal about the quality of consciousness at each stage and any insights that emerged.

Exercise 4: Cauldron Cultivation

Purpose: To establish and strengthen the energetic cauldrons in the three dantians.

Steps:

1. Begin in a seated meditation posture with relaxed, deep breathing.

2. Lower Dantian (10 minutes):

- Place attention about 1.5 inches below your navel and 1/3 of the way into your body.

- Visualize a cauldron forming in this space—traditionally seen as three-legged, round, and made of gold.

   - With each inhale, imagine gathering qi into this cauldron.

   - With each exhale, feel the qi being "cooked" and refined.

   - Notice sensations of warmth, fullness, or vibration.

3. Middle Dantian (10 minutes):

   - Shift attention to your heart center in the middle of your chest.

   - Visualize a red cauldron forming here.

   - Breathe into this space, feeling how it responds differently than the lower center.

   - Notice emotions and qualities of consciousness that arise.

4. Upper Dantian (10 minutes):

   - Move attention to the space between your eyebrows and slightly inside the head.

   - Visualize a luminous purple/white cauldron forming here.

   - Breathe gently while maintaining awareness of this center.

   - Notice qualities of clarity, spaciousness, or insight.

5. Integration (5 minutes):

   - Finally, bring awareness to all three cauldrons simultaneously.

   - Feel the relationship between them, noticing any communication or energy flow.

6. Record your experiences, noting which cauldron felt most accessible and which most challenging.

Exercise 5: Emptiness Contemplation

Purpose: To experience progressive degrees of emptiness and its relationship to consciousness.

Steps:

1. Find a comfortable meditation posture in a quiet environment.

2. Begin with 5 minutes of following your natural breath to settle the mind.

3. First level (5 minutes):

   - Contemplate a physical object in front of you.

   - Recognize that despite its apparent solidity, it is mostly empty space at the atomic level.

   - Feel this perception of solidity dissolving into awareness of space.

4. Second level (5 minutes):

   - Close your eyes and observe your thoughts as they arise.

   - Notice how each thought appears from emptiness and dissolves back into emptiness.

   - Recognize the space between thoughts as the same emptiness from which they emerge.

5. Third level (5 minutes):

   - Shift attention to the one who is observing—your sense of being a separate self.

   - Investigate: What is this awareness that knows both thoughts and emptiness?

   - Allow even this sense of a separate observer to relax and open.

6. Final phase (10 minutes):

   - Rest in the recognition that emptiness and awareness are not two separate things.

   - Experience consciousness as both empty of inherent existence and luminously present.

- Notice how this realization affects your sense of identity and relationship to experience.

7. Afterward, walk slowly for 5 minutes, maintaining this awareness of empty luminosity while moving in the world.

8. Journal about your experience, particularly noting any resistance or insights that emerged.

Journal Reflection

Contemplate: What symbols in Taoist alchemy resonate most with you, and why? What do they represent for you personally on physical, energetic, and spiritual levels?

Your Reflection:

_____

Practice Tracker

Use this table to track your daily inner alchemy practices. Note the symbols, dantian focus, or stages explored and any shifts in awareness or sensation.

Date	Practice Focus (e.g., Fire & Water, Cauldron)	Duration	Notable Experiences

Choose one symbol per day and reflect on its meaning for you:
- Cauldron
- Furnace
- Lead
- Gold
- Elixir

For each, write what it represents physically, energetically, and spiritually.

Cauldron

Physical Level:

_____

Energetic Level:

_____

Spiritual Level:

_____

Furnace

Physical Level:

_____

Energetic Level:

_____

Spiritual Level:

_____

Lead

Physical Level:

_____

Energetic Level:

_____

Spiritual Level:

_____

Gold

Physical Level:

_____

Energetic Level:

_____

Spiritual Level:

_____

Elixir

Physical Level:

_____

Energetic Level:

_____

Spiritual Level:

_____

Fire and Water Balancing Log

Reflect on your experience regulating fire and water energies (heart and kidneys):

Date	Balance Observed	Imbalance or Insight

Shen Fusion Journal

Document your experience in the stages of Shen fusion. Note how your awareness shifted, what arose in each stage, and how you perceived emptiness.

1. Gathering Shen:

_____

2. Refining Shen:

_____

3. Fusing Shen:

_____

4. Shen Returning to Emptiness:

_____

In the journey of spiritual cultivation, returning to the source represents the ultimate homecoming—a conscious reunion with our primordial nature. This chapter explores the profound practices of cultivating emptiness, witnessing Wuji (the unmanifested), and achieving Tao-realization through stillness. These ancient Taoist approaches offer pathways to transcend the limitations of ordinary perception and experience the boundless reality of our true nature.

Cultivating Emptiness

Emptiness (xu) in Taoist practice is not a nihilistic void, but rather a spacious awareness free from the clutter of conceptual thinking and attachment. When we cultivate emptiness, we create the internal conditions necessary for spontaneous harmony with the Tao.

The Taodejing reminds us: "We shape clay into a pot, but it is the emptiness inside that makes it useful." Similarly, our consciousness becomes most powerful when cleared of obstructions. Emptiness is not the absence of experience but the open field in which all experiences arise and dissolve.

Through the cultivation of emptiness, practitioners develop a profound receptivity to the subtle energies and wisdom of the universe. The mind becomes like a clear mirror, reflecting reality without distortion or bias. This state of inner clarity allows for direct perception of the Tao's workings in all phenomena.

Emptiness practice involves systematically releasing attachment to thoughts, emotions, and sensory experiences. By observing how these phenomena arise and pass away without clinging to them, we gradually discover the spacious awareness that remains constant amidst all changes.

Exercises for Cultivating Emptiness

Exercise 1: Clearing the Vessel

1. Sit in a comfortable position with your spine erect.

2. Bring awareness to your breath, allowing it to become smooth and natural.

3. Scan your body from head to toe, releasing any tension you encounter.

4. Notice thoughts as they arise, acknowledging them without judgment.

5. Visualize each thought as a cloud passing through the vast sky of your awareness.

6. As thoughts dissolve, allow your attention to rest in the spaciousness between thoughts.

7. Gradually extend the duration of resting in this mental spaciousness.

8. Practice for 15-20 minutes daily, gradually increasing to 30 minutes.

Exercise 2: The Water Bowl Practice

1. Place a bowl of water on a stable surface before you.

2. Sit comfortably and gaze at the surface of the water.

3. Allow your breathing to become subtle and even.

4. Observe how the water's surface reflects its surroundings without alteration.

5. Contemplate how your mind, when still, can reflect reality with similar clarity.

6. If the water is disturbed, notice how reflections become distorted—similar to how thoughts disturb perception.

7. As the water settles, allow your mind to settle in the same way.

8. Practice maintaining this still, reflective quality of mind for 10-15 minutes.

Exercise 3: Dissolving Boundaries Meditation

1. Begin in a seated meditation posture in a quiet environment.

2. Focus on your breathing until the mind becomes relatively calm.

3. Gradually expand your awareness to include the space around your body.

4. Feel the boundary between your body and the surrounding space becoming permeable.

5. Notice the sensations at this boundary, allowing them to soften and dissolve.

6. Experience your consciousness expanding beyond the confines of your physical form.

7. Rest in the experience of spaciousness that transcends the separation between self and environment.

8. When ready, gently return to normal awareness and reflect on the experience.

Witnessing Wuji (the unmanifested)

Wuji represents the primordial state of undifferentiated potential that precedes all manifestation. It is the unmanifested source from which the manifest universe emerges. In Taoist cosmology, Wuji gives rise to Taiji (the supreme ultimate), which then generates the interplay of yin and yang, eventually manifesting as the ten thousand things.

Witnessing Wuji is not an intellectual understanding but a direct experiential recognition of the unlimited potential that lies beneath all forms. This witness consciousness enables practitioners to perceive the unborn nature of reality—the ground of being prior to differentiation.

The practice involves a profound letting go of all constructs and categories, allowing consciousness to rest in its most fundamental state. From this perspective, the practitioner realizes that all phenomena are temporary expressions of the inexhaustible source. This recognition brings a profound freedom and release from the limitations of conditioned existence.

As the Zhuangzi states: "The Perfect Man uses his mind like a mirror—going after nothing, welcoming nothing, responding but not storing." This mirror-like quality of consciousness reflects the witness state that can perceive Wuji.

Exercises for Witnessing Wuji

Exercise 1: Tracing Back to the Source

1. Sit in meditation with your eyes softly closed.

2. Bring attention to any present experience—a thought, emotion, or sensation.

3. Ask yourself: "From where does this experience arise?"

4. Follow this experience back to its source in consciousness.

5. Continue this inquiry with each new arising, always tracing back to the source.

6. Notice the space of awareness that precedes all experiences.

7. Rest in this primordial awareness without attaching to any content that arises within it.

8. Practice for 20-30 minutes, gradually deepening your ability to rest at the source.

Exercise 2: The Gateway of Nonbeing

1. Begin in a comfortable seated position.

2. Focus on the pause between exhalation and inhalation.

3. Experience this pause as a doorway into nonbeing.

4. With each breath cycle, linger slightly longer in this threshold space.

5. Notice how this pause reflects the Wuji state—potential without manifestation.

6. Allow your consciousness to rest in this unmanifested state.

7. As you continue breathing naturally, maintain awareness of this gateway between being and nonbeing.

8. Practice for 15-20 minutes, gradually extending the time as your capacity develops.

Exercise 3: Dissolving into the Unborn

1. Sit in silent meditation in a darkened room.

2. Focus on the darkness before you, allowing your eyes to softly relax.

3. Perceive the darkness not as an absence of light but as the womb of all potential.

4. Feel your sense of separate self gradually dissolving into this infinite field.

5. Notice how forms and boundaries lose their solidity in this experience.

6. Rest in the recognition that your true nature is inseparable from this unmanifested ground.

7. Experience yourself as both the witness of and identical with this primordial state.

8. When complete, slowly return to ordinary awareness, retaining the insight of your essential nature.

Tao-realization in Stillness

Stillness (jing) in Taoist practice is not merely the absence of movement but a profound alignment with the unchanging essence that permeates all change. It is within deep stillness that the Tao reveals itself most directly. As the Taodejing advises: "Be still like a mountain and flow like a great river."

Tao-realization through stillness occurs when the practitioner's consciousness becomes so profoundly quiet that it merges with the silent source of all being. In this state, the artificial boundary between observer and observed dissolves, revealing the non-dual nature of reality.

The paradox of stillness is that it contains within it all movement, just as silence contains all sound. By cultivating absolute stillness, the practitioner discovers the living presence of the Tao that animates all phenomena while remaining eternally unmoved at its core.

This practice leads to what the Taoists call "action without action" (wei wu wei)—the ability to respond spontaneously and appropriately to life's circumstances without the interference of egoic striving. All action emerges organically from the still center, in perfect harmony with the natural unfolding of events.

Exercises for Tao-realization in Stillness

Exercise 1: Mountain Meditation

1. Sit with your spine straight, embodying the quality of a mountain.

2. Feel your body becoming heavy and immovable, rooted deeply in the earth.

3. Allow external movements and sounds to pass around you without disturbing your stillness.

4. Experience your breath as the gentle wind moving across the mountain's surface.

5. Thoughts and emotions become like changing weather patterns—observed but not affecting the mountain's essential nature.

6. Deepen into the unwavering presence at your core, beyond all transient experiences.

7. Rest in the recognition that true stillness persists through all changes and movements.

8. Practice for 25-30 minutes, cultivating increasingly profound levels of stillness.

Exercise 2: The Unmoving Center

1. Begin standing in the Wuji posture (feet shoulder-width apart, knees slightly bent, spine aligned).

2. Place your hands over your lower dantian (area below navel).

3. Slowly move your upper body in gentle circular motions.

4. As you move, maintain awareness of the still point at your center.

5. Gradually decrease the size of your movements while increasing awareness of stillness.

6. Eventually allow all external movement to cease, while experiencing the profound stillness at your core.

7. Notice how this stillness is not static but vibrant with life and potential.

8. Practice for 15-20 minutes, alternating between movement and stillness.

Exercise 3: Listening to Silence

1. Find a relatively quiet place for meditation.

2. Sit comfortably with eyes closed or softly focused.

3. First, bring attention to the various sounds in your environment.

4. Gradually shift your attention from the sounds themselves to the silence between and beneath the sounds.

5. As your attention deepens, perceive the field of silence that contains all sounds.

6. Allow your consciousness to merge with this all-encompassing silence.

7. Experience how this silence is not merely the absence of sound but the living presence of the Tao.

8. Rest in this silent awareness for 20-30 minutes, letting insights arise naturally from this state.

Integration: The Continuous Return

The practices of cultivating emptiness, witnessing Wuji, and realizing the Tao through stillness are not separate endeavors but interconnected aspects of the same journey. Together, they facilitate what the Taoists call "returning to the source"—the conscious reunification with our original nature.

This return is not a one-time achievement but a continuous process of remembering and realigning with the Tao. Each moment offers an opportunity to release attachment, witness the unmanifested ground of being, and embody stillness in action.

As you integrate these practices into daily life, you may notice a gradual transformation in your perception and experience. The world appears increasingly as a seamless expression of the source, with each phenomenon revealing its intimate connection to the whole. This vision of interconnected wholeness is the hallmark of Tao-realization.

Remember that returning to the source is not an escape from the world but a profound reengagement with it from the perspective of unity consciousness. From this recognition, compassion and wisdom flow naturally, and life becomes an effortless expression of the Tao's spontaneous unfolding.

Through dedicated practice and sincere inquiry, the journey of returning to the source culminates in the realization that we have never truly been separate from it. As the ancient Taoist texts remind us: "The Tao is near, but people seek it far away."

Workbook: Returning to the Source (Xu)

Journal Reflection

Contemplate: Reflect on what 'returning to the source' means to you. How do you relate to the concept of emptiness or the unmanifested (Wuji)? How does stillness show up in your current life or practice?

Your Reflection:

_____

Practice Tracker

Use this table to track your daily practices for cultivating emptiness, witnessing Wuji, and Tao-realization in stillness.

Date	Practice Focus (Emptiness, Wuji, Stillness)	Duration	Insights / Experiences

Emptiness Practice Log

Clearing the Vessel

Describe your experience with this practice:

Water Bowl Practice

Describe your experience with this practice:

Dissolving Boundaries Meditation

Describe your experience with this practice:

Wuji Witnessing Practice Log

Tracing Back to the Source

Describe your experience with this practice:

The Gateway of Nonbeing

Describe your experience with this practice:

Dissolving into the Unborn

Describe your experience with this practice:

Stillness and Tao-realization Log

Mountain Meditation

Describe your experience with this practice:

The Unmoving Center

Describe your experience with this practice:

Listening to Silence

Describe your experience with this practice:

"The Tao that can be told is not the eternal Tao.
The name that can be named is not the eternal name."
— Lao Tzu, Tao Te Ching

The journey of Taoist cultivation is not meant to end on the meditation cushion. The true power of the Tao is revealed when its principles flow seamlessly into every aspect of our daily existence. This chapter explores the final transformation on the path: the dissolution of boundaries between formal practice and everyday life.

When we first begin our Taoist practice, we create a distinct separation—there is "practice time" and there is "regular life." We may meditate in the morning, practice qigong at noon, and study ancient texts in the evening. These are beautiful and necessary steps on the path. Yet the highest achievement is not perfecting these practices but transcending the very notion that practice is something separate from life itself.

In this chapter, we will explore three essential aspects of living the Tao: integration into daily life, the cultivation of compassion and humility, and the art of dissolving boundaries between practice and life. Through practical exercises and contemplative inquiries, you will discover how to embody the Tao in each breath, step, and interaction—transforming ordinary moments into expressions of the extraordinary wisdom that has guided seekers for thousands of years.

Part I: Integration into Daily Life

Understanding Integration

Integration means weaving the principles of the Tao—simplicity, naturalness, non-contention, and spontaneity—into the fabric of ordinary existence. It means that washing dishes becomes as profound as formal meditation, that dealing with a difficult colleague becomes an opportunity to practice non-resistance, and that choosing what to eat becomes an exercise in mindfulness and harmony.

True integration happens when we no longer need to remind ourselves to "be Taoist" in our actions. Instead, the principles of the Tao begin to express themselves naturally through us, like water finding its course downhill. The ancient masters described this as "acting without action" (wu-wei)—not forced behavior, but natural, appropriate response arising from a deep alignment with the Tao.

"The perfect man employs his mind as a mirror. It grasps nothing, it refuses nothing. It receives but does not keep."
— Zhuangzi

Exercises for Daily Integration

Exercise 1: Mindful Transitions

Purpose: To bring awareness to the thresholds between different activities in your day.

Steps:

1. Identify 3-5 major transitions in your daily routine (e.g., waking up, leaving home, starting work, ending work, preparing for sleep).
2. For one week, pause for three conscious breaths at each transition point.
3. During these breaths, ask yourself: "What energy am I carrying from the previous activity? What energy would serve me best in the next activity?"
4. Consciously release any tension, hurry, or residual emotions that don't serve the next phase of your day.
5. Move into the new activity with fresh awareness, as if it were the only thing in the world.
6. At the end of each day, journal about what you noticed during these transition moments.

Exercise 2: Tao of Ordinary Tasks

Purpose: To discover profound presence in routine activities.

Steps:

1. Select one ordinary task you perform daily (dishes, showering, commuting, preparing food, etc.).
2. For the next seven days, approach this task as sacred practice.
3. Before beginning, take a moment to quiet your mind and set an intention to be fully present.
4. Engage all your senses—notice textures, sounds, smells, visual details.
5. Slow down the activity by 20% from your usual pace.

6. When your mind wanders (and it will), gently bring it back to the sensory experience.
7. Notice any resistance, boredom, or hurry that arises, without judgment.
8. After completing the task, take a moment to appreciate having had the opportunity to perform it.
9. In your journal, record any insights that emerged during these "ordinary" moments.

Exercise 3: Wu-Wei Decision Making

Purpose: To practice "effortless action" in daily choices.

Steps:

1. For the next three days, before making any decision (small or large), pause.
2. Take three deep breaths to center yourself.
3. Ask yourself: "What would be the most natural course of action here? What would require the least force or strain?"
4. Notice if there are multiple possible paths that feel equally natural and unforced.
5. Make your choice based on what feels most aligned with ease and harmony.
6. After implementing your decision, reflect: Did it flow naturally? Did it create harmony or discord?
7. Record your observations about which decisions felt most aligned with wu-wei principles.

Part II: Compassion, Humility, Presence

The Virtues of the Tao

While the Tao itself is beyond all qualities and attributes, those who align with it naturally express certain virtues. Chief among these are compassion (ci), humility (qian), and presence (zai). These are not moral imperatives imposed from outside but natural expressions of one who has realized their unity with all things.

Compassion in Taoism is not merely feeling sorry for others; it is recognizing that there is no fundamental separation between self and other. The suffering of another is, in a real sense, our own suffering. Humility arises not from thinking less of oneself but from releasing the need to assert the ego at all. And presence—perhaps the most essential quality—means being fully available to life as it unfolds, without the distortions of excessive thinking about past or future.

"When I let go of what I am, I become what I might be. When I let go of what I have, I receive what I need."
— Lao Tzu

Exercise 4: The Compassion Practice

Purpose: To develop universal compassion through recognizing shared humanity.

Steps:

1. Begin with 5-10 minutes of quiet breathing meditation to center yourself.
2. Bring to mind someone you care deeply about. Feel your natural warmth and care for them.
3. Silently repeat: "Just like me, this person wishes to be happy. Just like me, this person knows suffering."
4. Now bring to mind an acquaintance—someone you neither like nor dislike. Repeat the same contemplation.
5. Finally, bring to mind someone difficult—a person you struggle with. Again repeat: "Just like me, this person wishes to be happy. Just like me, this person knows suffering."
6. Notice any resistance that arises and allow it to be present without judgment.
7. Extend your awareness to all beings everywhere: "Just like me, all beings wish to be happy. Just like me, all beings know suffering."
8. Rest in the spacious awareness that holds all beings in compassion.
9. Journal about what you discovered, especially regarding the difficult person.

Exercise 5: Humility of Not-Knowing

Purpose: To cultivate the freedom that comes from releasing certainty.

Steps:

1. For one week, maintain an "I don't know" journal.
2. Each evening, write down at least three instances during the day when you:
    - Pretended to know something you weren't certain about
    - Argued for your position as the "right" one
    - Made assumptions without adequate information
    - Judged someone or something hastily

3. For each instance, write what it would have felt like to simply say (internally or externally): "I don't know."
4. The following day, practice saying "I don't know" or "I'm not sure" when appropriate.
5. Notice the physical sensation of releasing the need to know, to be right, or to have an answer.
6. At the end of the week, reflect on how this practice affected your interactions and peace of mind.

Exercise 6: The Bell of Presence

Purpose: To develop consistent present-moment awareness throughout the day.

Steps:

1. Set a gentle alarm or "bell of mindfulness" to sound randomly 5-7 times throughout your day.
2. When the bell sounds, pause whatever you're doing (if safe to do so).
3. Take three conscious breaths.
4. Ask yourself: "Where am I right now? What is happening in this moment?"
5. Notice three things you can see, two things you can hear, and one sensation in your body.
6. Check in with your emotional state without trying to change it.
7. Identify if you were mentally "time traveling" to past or future before the bell.
8. Continue your activity with renewed presence.
9. At the end of the day, reflect on what patterns you noticed about when you tend to lose presence.

Part III: Dissolving Boundaries Between Practice and Life

The Seamless Tao

The final transformation on the Taoist path is the recognition that there was never any real boundary between "practice" and "life." The artificial separation we created was merely a teaching tool—like the finger pointing to the moon, necessary at first but ultimately to be transcended.

In this realization, every breath becomes meditation, every interaction becomes an opportunity for compassion, every challenge becomes a teacher. The sacred and the ordinary reveal themselves as one continuous reality. The Taoist practitioner reaches the stage where they no longer "do" Taoism—they simply live, and that living is the perfect expression of the Tao.

"The Tao is near and people seek it far away."
— Mencius

Exercise 7: Sacred Encounters

Purpose: To recognize the extraordinary within ordinary encounters.

Steps:

1. For one week, approach each person you meet as if they were a teacher sent specifically for you.
2. Before each significant interaction, silently ask yourself: "What might this person have to teach me?"
3. During the interaction, listen more than you speak. Notice subtle wisdom in their words, even if presented simply.
4. Pay attention to your reactions—moments of resonance, resistance, judgment, or inspiration.
5. After the interaction, take a moment to reflect: "What did I learn from this encounter?"
6. Each evening, record the most significant "teaching" you received that day from an ordinary encounter.
7. At the end of the week, review your notes and identify patterns in what life has been trying to show you.

Exercise 8: The Formless Practice

Purpose: To experience practice without formal structure.

Steps:

1. Set aside one day (or at least half a day) for this exercise.
2. On this day, make no formal plans for spiritual practice—no meditation time, no qigong, no specific readings.
3. Begin the day with the intention: "Today, I will discover how the Tao expresses itself naturally through my life."

4. Move through your day with heightened awareness, but without structuring "practice time."
5. Notice moments when:
   - You naturally become silent and present
   - Your breath deepens without conscious effort
   - Compassion arises spontaneously
   - You find yourself in a state of flow
   - Wisdom emerges without seeking it
6. At day's end, reflect: "How did the Tao express itself through me today without formal practice?"
7. Consider which elements of formless practice you might incorporate into your daily life.

Exercise 9: The Thread of Awareness

Purpose: To maintain continuous awareness throughout diverse activities.

Steps:

1. Choose one full day for this practice.
2. Select a simple physical "anchor" for awareness—such as the sensation of your feet touching the ground, your breath, or your hands.
3. Set an intention to maintain awareness of this anchor throughout the day, regardless of what activities you engage in.
4. As you move from activity to activity, maintain this thread of awareness as a constant.
5. When you notice you've lost the thread, simply reconnect with your anchor without judgment.
6. Notice how this continuous awareness transforms various activities—from the mundane to the complex.
7. Observe how maintaining this thread helps dissolve the sense of "switching" between different modes of being.
8. At day's end, reflect on when the thread was strongest and when it was most challenging to maintain.
9. Consider how this practice reveals the artificial nature of boundaries we create in our experience.

Conclusion: The Ongoing Journey

Living the Tao is not a destination but a continually unfolding journey. Each moment offers a fresh opportunity to align more deeply with the natural way. The practices and exercises in this chapter are not meant to be completed and set aside but revisited regularly as your understanding evolves.

Remember that the highest teaching of the Tao is extraordinarily simple: Live naturally, in harmony with your true nature and the flow of life. All techniques, practices, and philosophies are merely temporary scaffolding to help you remember what, at some level, you have always known.

As you continue on this path, be patient with yourself. There will be days of profound clarity and days of seeming regression. Both are part of the natural rhythm of growth. The Tao embraces all experiences without preference, and so can you.

May your journey of living the Tao bring increasing freedom, joy, and harmony— not just to yourself, but to all whose lives you touch.

"The further you go, the less you know."
— Lao Tzu

Reflection Questions

Consider these questions:

1. In what areas of your life do you still maintain a separation between "practice" and "regular life"?
2. Which of the three virtues—compassion, humility, or presence—comes most naturally to you? Which requires more conscious cultivation?
3. What would your life look like if you fully embodied the principles of the Tao in every moment?
4. How has your understanding of what it means to "practice" the Tao evolved since beginning this journey?
5. What is one small step you can take today to bring more alignment between your inner cultivation and your outer expression?

Remember: The true measure of understanding is not what you know about the Tao, but how you live it.

Journal Reflection

Contemplate: How do you currently distinguish between your spiritual practice and your daily life? Inwhat ways could those boundaries begin to dissolve?

Your Reflection:

Practice Tracker

Use this table to track your daily Living-the-Tao practices, focusing on integration, virtues, and seamless awareness.

Date	Practice Focus (e.g., Integration, Compassion, Wu-Wei)	Insight or Teaching	Integration into Daily Life

Integration Practices Log

Mindful Transitions

Describe your experience with this practice:

Tao of Ordinary Tasks

Describe your experience with this practice:

Wu-Wei Decision Making

Describe your experience with this practice:

Taoist Virtues Practice Log

The Compassion Practice

Describe your experience with this practice:

Humility of Not-Knowing

Describe your experience with this practice:

The Bell of Presence

Describe your experience with this practice:

Seamless Tao Practices Log

Sacred Encounters

Describe your experience with this practice:

_____

The Formless Practice

Describe your experience with this practice:

_____

The Thread of Awareness

Describe your experience with this practice:

_____

Final Reflection Questions

1. In what areas of your life do you still maintain a separation between 'practice' and 'regular life'?

_____

2. Which of the three virtues—compassion, humility, or presence—comes most naturally to you? Which requires more conscious cultivation?

_____

3. What would your life look like if you fully embodied the principles of the Tao in every moment?

_____

4. How has your understanding of what it means to 'practice' the Tao evolved since beginning this journey?

_____

5. What is one small step you can take today to bring more alignment between your inner cultivation and your outer expression?

_____

Chapter 13: The Journey Continues – Walking the Way

"A good traveler has no fixed plans, and is not intent on arriving."
— Lao Tzu, *Tao Te Ching*

You have now walked the winding path through **Nei Gong**, **Shen Gong**, and **Nei Dan**—a journey that led from grounding the body, to awakening spirit, to dissolving the self in the vastness of the Tao.

And yet, here you are—not at an end, but at a beginning.

The Seeds You've Planted

Through every breath, posture, and meditation, you have cultivated not just energy, but awareness. You have built a reservoir of Qi in your Dantian, refined the clarity of your Shen, and opened the inner doors to Emptiness (Xu)—the silent, formless field in which all things arise and return.

These are not small accomplishments.

Even if your progress felt subtle at times, even if there were doubts or dry spells, know this: the seeds are alive within you. The Tao does not bloom on demand—it emerges organically, in its own rhythm, in stillness and in flow.

The Path is Now Yours

At this point, there is no need to memorize more techniques or chase after exotic experiences. The real teaching now lies in living.

- In breathing with awareness as you walk through a busy day
- In listening deeply when someone speaks
- In responding to difficulty not with resistance, but with presence
- In letting go of control and trusting the current beneath the surface of things

These are the alchemical fires now. These are the crucibles.

What you once practiced in stillness, you are now invited to live in motion.

You Are the Elixir

The goal of Taoist alchemy was never merely to accumulate power or attain mystical states. The true transformation happens when you **become** the elixir—the one who embodies harmony, lightness, depth, and flow. Not to impress, not to perform, but simply to be.

The Immortal Embryo, the Light Body, the Shen returning to Emptiness—these are not mystical achievements to grasp, but natural unfoldings when the practitioner no longer stands in the way of what already is.

You are not separate from the Tao. You never were.

Keep Returning

Even now, you may forget. You may find yourself back in old patterns or distractions. This, too, is part of the way.

Return.

Return to your breath.
Return to the Dantian.
Return to the quiet awareness behind all experiences.

Each return is a blessing. Each moment is new.

Parting Words

The Tao is not a place to reach.
It is the rhythm of your life when lived in harmony with your true nature.
May your days be filled with stillness, your heart with compassion, and your steps with presence.
May you live lightly, love deeply, and flow freely.
And when in doubt—breathe, soften, and return.

You are already home.

"The sage travels all day yet never leaves home."
— *Tao Te Ching*

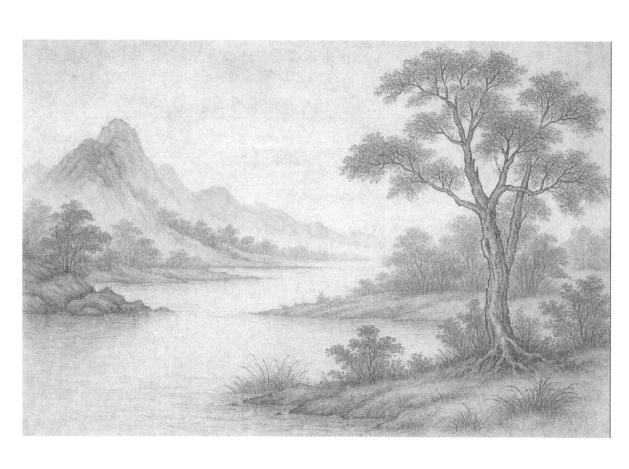

Made in the USA
Middletown, DE
01 May 2025

75008001R00126